MILD TRAUMATIC BRAIN INJURY

A Therapy and Resource Manual

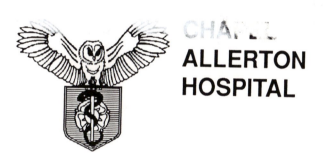

CHAPEL
ALLERTON
HOSPITAL

POSTGRADUATE
LIBRARY

Neurogenic Communication Disorders Series

SERIES EDITOR

Leonard L. LaPointe, Ph.D.

Developmental Motor Speech Disorders
Michael A. Crary

Cognitive-Communicative Abilities Following Brain Injury: A Functional Approach
Leila L. Hartley

Pediatric Traumatic Brain Injury: Proactive Intervention
Jean L. Blosser and Roberta DePompei

Mild Traumatic Brain Injury: A Therapy and Resource Manual
Betsy S. Green, Kristin M. Stevens, and Tracey D. W. Wolfe

Mild Traumatic Brain Injury

A Therapy and Resource Manual

Neurogenic Communication Disorder Series

Betsy S. Green, M.A., CCC-SLP
Kristin M. Stevens, M.A.T., CCC-SLP
Tracey D.W. Wolfe, M.S., CCC-SLP

Therapeutic Rehabilitation Center
Farmington Hills, Michigan

SINGULAR PUBLISHING GROUP, INC.
SAN DIEGO . LONDON

Singular Publishing Group, Inc.
401 West "A" Street, Suite 325
San Diego, California 92101-7904

Singular Publishing Ltd.
19 Compton Terrace
London, N1 2UN, UK

e-mail: singpub@mail.cerfnet.com
Website: http://www.singpub.com

Typeset in 11/13 Bookman Book by So Cal Graphics
Printed in the United States of America by McNaughton and Gunn

Library of Congress Cataloging-in-Publication Data

Green, Betsy S.
    Mild traumatic brain injury : a therapy and resource manual /
Betsy S. Green, Kristin M. Stevens, Tracey D. W. Wolfe.
        p.   cm
    Includes bibliographical references and index.
    ISBN 1–56593–827–5
    1. Brain damage—Patients—Rehabilitation.   2. Brain—Wounds and
injuries—Patients—Rehabilitation.   3. Cognition disorders—Patients—
Rehabilitation.   I. Stevens, Kristin M.   II. Wolfe,
Tracey D. W.   III. Title.
    [DNLM: 1. Brain Injuries—rehabilitation.   2. Brain Injuries—
diagnosis.   3. Speech Therapy.   4. Language Therapy. WL354 G795m
1997]
RC387.5.G74   1997
616.8'043—dc21
DNLM/DLC
for Library of Congress
                                                                    97-25314
                                                                    CIP

Contents

3 TREATMENT OF MILD-TO-MODERATE TRAUMATIC BRAIN INJURY

4 TREATING COMPLEX ATTENTION IMPAIRMENTS

5 TREATING FUNCTIONAL AND PROSPECTIVE MEMORY IMPAIRMENTS

6 TREATING WORD RETRIEVAL AND THOUGHT FORMULATION IMPAIRMENTS

Foreword

The brain is a marvelous thing. It has been called the only human organ capable of studying itself. Although the metaphoric heart has been rhapsodized much more frequently in song and sonnet, the brain and its peculiar music has met increasing attention, not only popularly, but notably from researchers, scholars, educators, and clinicians who must deal with attempts to understand it. In fact, in the United States, the commitment to understanding the brain and its disorders is reflected in the highest policy levels of the government, and the White House Office of Science and Technology Policy focused this attention in a report entitled, "Maximizing Human Potential: Decade of the Brain 1990–2000."

When the human nervous system goes awry, the cost is enormous. The direct and indirect economic impact of brain disorders in the United States has been estimated to be over 400 billion dollars. It is impossible to measure the toll that brain disorders exact in terms of human agony from survivors and their families. Each disruption of delicate neural balance can cause problems in moving, sensing, eating, thinking, and a rich array of human behaviors. Certainly not the least of these are those unique human attributes involved in communication. To speak, to understand, to write, to read, to remember, to create, to calculate, to plan, to reason, and myriad other cognitive and communicative acts are the sparks and essence of human interaction. When they are lost or impaired, isolation can result, or at the very least, quality of life can be compromised. This series is about the many conditions that arise from brain or nervous system damage that can affect these human cognitive and communicative functions. But it is not only an attempt to understand the disruption and negative effects of neurogenic disorders. As well, the authors in this series will show that there is a positive side. Rehabilitation, relearning, intervention, recovery, adjustment, acceptance, and reintegration are the rewards to be extracted from challenge. There is no shortage of these features in this series. Frustrations and barriers can be redeemed by recovery and small victories. The works in the Singular Neurogenic Communication Disorders Series address both the obstacles and the triumphs.

This book is a bit of a departure in format and content from the others in the series. Green, Stevens, and Wolfe are experienced clinicians who have a good deal of experience in setting up and implementing clinical management plans for people with traumatic brain injury (TBI). Their combined experience has led to insights into what practicing clinicians need to help solve the intervention riddles of this most challenging population. The need for a therapy and resource manual on clinical management of the cognitive and communicative impairment, disability, and handicap of people with TBI has often been articulated by clinicians. New clinicians especially have voiced the need for practical guidance on dealing with the web of clinical responsibilities these clients present. This book goes a long way toward fulfilling this need. The manual focuses on mild-to-moderate levels of cognitive and communication problems of people with TBI. Although this level of severity is the target population, the book contains material that may be extracted or adapted for those who are more severely involved. Not very much material or information is available for the mildly to moderately involved, however, and one of the strengths of this manual is its focus on this segment of the severity range. The targeted age span is adolescence and adulthood, although again some of the suggestions in the manual might be found useful for survivors of TBI younger than teenagers, if the clinician using the manual makes age-appropriate adjustments of the material.

The manual is, first and foremost, a therapy and reference manual. As such, it is not prescriptive for each individual with TBI who may be encountered, but it surely can serve as a guide that can be adapted and customized to the idiosyncratic needs of each client. Even the casual reader will discover that this work is a mother lode of clinical help. It is full of sample letters for addressing academic, vocational, reimbursement, and treatment authorization issues. The reader will find pages of material on suggested formats and content for client interviews, checklists, and forms and surveys for organizing and categorizing clinical observations. Chapter 1 presents an overview of the diversified roles of the speech-language pathologist in confronting the challenges of TBI, with particular emphasis on our role with family members and other professionals on the rehabilitative and educational team. Chapter 2 presents specific guidelines for assessment of mild-to-moderate TBI. Included in this chapter are sample evaluation segments and information on assessment devices and standardized tests. Suggestions on assessment planning are coupled with strategies for evaluating specific cognitive and communication domains.

The heart of this manual is the corpus of suggestions and materials on treatment contained in Chapters 3 through 8. Chapter 3 discusses development of a treatment plan and a rationale for the selection of treatment targets. In Chapters 4–8, a separate cognitive-communicative domain is defined and discussed (complex attention, functional and prospective memory, word retrieval and thought formulation, auditory and visual information processing, executive functions). Each of these domains is discussed relative to the functional implications of the impairment. Then very specific therapy tasks and compensatory strategies are outlined along with home practice tasks and suggestions for families. In the final chapter, details of clinical management are addressed with suggestions on therapy documentation, transition and discharge from therapy, and ideas for follow-up. Clinicians will benefit deeply from this section of the manual. The myriad functional and creative tasks that are presented here, along with the scores of additional resources and ideas that are directly related to therapy, will make this book an indispensable resource for clinicians charged with the poignant responsibility of dealing with the cognitive-communicative problems that revolve around people who have been visited with the "silent epidemic" of traumatic brain injury.

Leonard L. LaPointe
Series Editor
Arizona State University

Preface

This reference and therapy manual was created to address the unique needs of adolescents and adults who have sustained mild-to-moderate traumatic brain injuries. Limited published therapy materials exist to meet the specific needs of these higher functioning, yet impaired individuals. Following an acquired mild-to-moderate traumatic brain injury (TBI), an individual's level of impairment may not be accurately determined or addressed due to the difficulty in evaluating and treating subtle, yet functionally significant deficits. In our opinion, a brain injury medically labeled "mild" or "moderate" can produce devastating effects in the lives of individuals who have previously led active, productive lifestyles. This is underscored by typical complaints and concerns expressed by our clients, such as, "I'm having difficulty concentrating," "I get easily distracted," "I don't feel organized," and "I can't seem to accomplish anything I start." Reported comments further indicate that clients with TBI have difficulty expressing their thoughts, understanding what others say to them, and recalling information they have heard or read. For example, clients often report, "I can't seem to say what I mean," "I lose my train of thought," "I can't remember what I read to share with others," and "This has eroded my confidence at work." Subtle complaints often become major concerns when these individuals attempt to manage their daily responsibilities and return to demanding jobs.

When reviewing the available statistical information provided by the National Brain Injury Association, Inc., one can easily be astonished by the frequency of head injury occurrence. Each year in the United States, 2 million people sustain a traumatic brain injury—one every 15 seconds. It has been estimated that TBI claims more than 56,000 lives annually (Kraus & McArthur, 1995), and approximately 373,000 individuals require hospitalization (Kraus & Sorenson, 1994).

According to McAllister (1994), a conservative estimate derived from epidemiological studies such as Whitman et al. (1984) and Rimel (1981) indicates that *mild* TBI accounts for one half to three quarters of all patients hospitalized with a brain injury. Furthermore, according to an epidemiological study by Kraus and Nourjah (1989), it is estimated that as many as four to five mild brain injuries occur for each one that results in hospitalization. Most individuals with *mild* TBI are seen on an outpatient basis and are sent home with the recommendations to briefly recuperate without formal rehabilitation and return to work and other daily responsibilities as soon as possible. Yet, as stated by Bennett (1992), "Attention and memory difficulties, while a common sequel of brain injury, are often underestimated with respect to their negative impact on running a household, returning to work, and re-entering school. Many activities require high levels of sustained and divided attention" (p 25). As these individuals attempt to resume their demanding responsibilities at home, work, or school, significant difficulties become increasingly evident, causing greater cognitive and emotional concern. As these deficits often interfere with maintaining relationships and completing once easily accomplished home, work, or school tasks, most clients begin to question their ability to continue to lead a full, productive life. After a considerable time delay, concern regarding their deteriorating psychological and cognitive status often leads them to seek additional professional assistance (Kay, 1986).

In working with numerous higher functioning clients, we have relied on our clinical judgment and investigation to develop assessment protocols and treatment tasks. Other than published articles describing typical complaints, symptoms, and characteristics, few therapy resources are available for clinicians to utilize in working with these challenging individuals, who require specialized treatment to meet their rehabilitation needs. In compiling this manual, it is our intention to provide reference information, treatment tasks, and resource ideas to both assist clinicians and encourage them to further explore and create useful and individualized therapy approaches when treating this challenging population.

Chapter 1, which discusses the diversified roles of the speech-language pathologist, is based on many years of clinical experience, "on-the-job training" to appreciate these various roles, and a collection of resource information gathered from conferences, colleagues, and publications. This essential component of the manual will enhance future clinicians' understanding of the many roles they need to fulfill and encourage current professionals to become more flexible and comfortable with defining their job responsibilities.

Chapter 2 provides essential evaluation information, designed to assist the clinician in best determining clients' skill strengths and limitations, choosing appropriate formal and informal assessment materials, documenting areas of skill breakdown, outlining treatment recommendations, and developing functional therapy goals. Additionally, an interview questionnaire, observation checklist, sample evaluation reports, and sample vocational recommendations are provided.

Chapters 3 through 8 provide functional therapy tasks and strategies targeting skills necessary for increased independence in the home and community. These tasks also embrace the objective of reintegration into the work setting and school environment. The tasks in each skill unit address limitations in the areas of complex attention, functional and prospective memory, word retrieval and thought formulation, information processing, and executive functioning. We suggest utilizing the sample tasks as structured therapy practice for clients, as well as for further documentation of skill breakdown to guide individualized treatment task planning. We provide descriptions of possible compensatory strategies and specific suggestions for further practice under each skill area to promote refinement of skills. This manual is targeted mainly for use with individuals with mild-to-moderate TBI; however, tasks may be utilized with individuals with a variety of other neurological disabilities.

The manual is designed as both a reference and therapy guide to assist speech-language pathologists in the evaluation and treatment of the cognitive and communicative problems of higher functioning individuals, who may have significant skill limitations. *We intend to offer information that will supplement your fundamental knowledge, provide a framework for your clinical approach, and provide specific therapeutic suggestions for ser-*

vicing this unique client population. In addition, we have carefully selected practical research-based resource materials and reference articles to supplement your knowledge and provide further sources of information. Articles listed in Chapter 1 were selected because they present fundamental information on TBI, which will assist you in expanding your knowledge base as a speech-language pathologist working with mild-to-moderate TBI. Resource articles in Chapter 2 provide information regarding assessment, and Chapter 3 lists sources of additional information specifically focusing on treatment and intervention issues.

Furthermore, to provide a foundation for understanding our approach to servicing this population, we subscribe to the well-accepted definition from the American Congress of Rehabilitation Medicine (Kay et al., 1993) reprinted on the following pages. This framework thoroughly defines and describes mild TBI and the resulting physical, cognitive, and behavioral changes, as well as the physiology of how this type of injury occurs.

Finally, throughout this manual, we refer to individuals we treat as "clients." We prefer this terminology because it implies an active, cooperative relationship between the clinician and individual, and this reflects our rehabilitation philosophy.

Betsy Green
Kris Stevens
Tracey Wolfe

Definition of Mild Traumatic Brain Injury[1]

DEFINITION

A patient with mild traumatic brain injury is a person who has had a traumatically induced physiological disruption of brain function, as manifested by **at least one** of the following:

1. any period of loss of consciousness;

2. any loss of memory for events immediately before or after the accident;

3. any alteration in mental state at the time of the accident (eg, feeling dazed, disoriented, or confused); and

4. focal neurological deficit(s) that may or may not be transient;

   but where the severity of the injury does not exceed the following:

   ■ loss of consciousness of approximately 30 minutes or less;

   ■ after 30 minutes, an initial Glasgow Coma Scale (GCS) of 13–15; and

   ■ posttraumatic amnesia (PTA) not greater than 24 hours.

COMMENTS

This definition includes: (1) the head being struck, (2) the head striking an object, and (3) the brain undergoing an acceleration/deceleration movement (ie, whiplash) without direct external trauma to the head. It excludes stroke, anoxia, tumor, encephalitis, etc.

---

[1] Reprinted with permission from Definition of Mild Traumatic Brain Injury by Thomas Kay and the Mild Traumatic Brain Injury Committee of the Head Injury Special Interst Group of the American Congress of Rehabilitation Medicine, 1993, pp. 86–87. *Journal of Head Trauma Rehabilitation, 8*(3). Aspen Publishers, Inc.

Computed tomography, magnetic resonance imaging electroencephalogram, or routine neurological evaluations may be normal. Due to the lack of medical emergency, or the realities of certain medical systems, some patients may not have the above factors medically documented in the acute stage. In such cases, it is appropriate to consider symptomatology that, when linked to a traumatic head injury, can suggest the existence of a mild traumatic brain injury.

SYMPTOMATOLOGY

The above criteria define the event of a mild traumatic brain injury. Symptoms of brain injury may or may not persist, for varying lengths of time, after such a neurological event. It should be recognized that patients with mild traumatic brain injury can exhibit persistent emotional, cognitive, behavioral, and physical symptoms, alone or in combination, which may produce a functional disability. These symptoms generally fall into one of the following categories, and are additional evidence that a mild traumatic brain injury has occurred:

1. physical symptoms of brain injury (eg, nausea, vomiting, dizziness, headache, blurred vision, sleep disturbance, quickness to fatigue, lethargy, or other sensory loss) that cannot be accounted for by peripheral injury or other causes;

2. cognitive deficits (eg, involving attention, concentration, perception, memory, speech/language, or executive functions) that cannot be completely accounted for by emotional state or other causes; and

3. behavioral change(s) and/or alterations in degree of emotional responsivity (eg, irritability, quickness to anger, disinhibition, or emotional lability) that cannot be accounted for by a psychological reaction to physical or emotional stress or other causes.

COMMENTS

Some patients may not become aware of, or admit, the extent of their symptoms until they attempt to return to normal functioning. In such cases, the evidence for mild traumatic brain injury must be reconstructed. Mild traumatic brain injury may also be overlooked in the face of more dramatic physical injury (eg, orthopedic or spinal cord injury). The constellation of symptoms has previously been referred to as minor head injury, postconcussive syndrome, traumatic head syndrome, traumatic cephalgia, post-brain injury syndrome and posttraumatic syndrome.

CONTRIBUTING AUTHORS

Thomas Kay, PhD, Senior Contributor
Douglas E. Harrington, PhD, Committee Chair
Richard Adams, MD
Thomas Anderson, MD
Sheldon Berrol, MD

Keith Cicerone, PhD
Cynthia Dahlberg, MA, CCC
Don Gerber, PhD
Richard Goka, MD
Preston Harley, PhD
Judy Hilt, RN
Lawrence Horn, MD
Donald Lehmkuhl, PhD
James Malec, PhD

ACKNOWLEDGMENTS

We wish to thank our colleagues, Barbara Hill, Debbie Fidge, and Dr. Russ Reeves, who continually offered their supportive encouragement and helpful assistance whenever needed. Additionally, we appreciate the ongoing assistance and positive feedback provided by Dr. Leonard LaPointe and Singular Publishing Group associates Candice Janco and Sandy Doyle.

We would also like to extend a special acknowledgment to our past and present clients, who continue to stimulate our creativity and challenge our knowledge, enabling us to grow as therapists and people.

Most importantly, we wish to extend our deepest gratitude to our husbands, Eric, Joe, and Eric, who inspire us with their humor, kindness, guidance, and love. They have expressed great pride in our pursuit of this exciting endeavor and we are continually amazed by their never-ending support.

DEDICATIONS

To my parents, who fostered in me a love for learning and showed me by their example how to truly have compassion for others. These gifts will always be with me. Thank you.

To my sweet, spirited Emma, who has broadened my concept of "communication" by speaking to my heart with her smiles, curiosity, sensitivity, and enthusiasm.
BSG

To my parents, whose love and support have been a constant in my life. Thank you for always encouraging my dreams and believing in my abilities. You are truly "the wind beneath my wings."
KMS

To my Dad, who through his own health concerns, taught me that being disabled does not mean you are unable. His spirit was admirable and I miss him.

To my Mom, who taught me that a strong will, determination, and compassion for others will best enable me to handle life's challenges. I am proud to be your daughter.
TDWW

CHAPTER 1

The Diversified Roles of the Speech-Language Pathologist

The speech-language pathologist working with individuals with mild-to-moderate traumatic brain injury (TBI) is required to fulfill a variety of professional roles. Although specialized training in cognitive and communicative processes provides much of the framework for several of these roles, clinicians often are not fully prepared to carry out each role described. Additionally, clinicians may be required to redefine their roles as part of a rehabilitation team in the current, ever changing healthcare environment. This section describes each of the important roles the authors have fulfilled when working with people with mild-to-moderate TBI.

EVALUATION, TREATMENT, AND INFORMATION SHARING

The most significant and time-consuming role of the speech-language pathologist in working with this population involves providing direct evaluation and functional treatment of individuals with mild-to-moderate TBI. Initial diagnostic assessment is completed using a variety of test protocols (listed in Chapter 2) to determine the client's current functioning and skill levels. The speech-language pathologist must evaluate the subtle, yet functionally significant, limitations associated with mild-to-moderate TBI. Cognitive-language skill areas addressed during assessment and treatment may include:

- Complex attention

- Functional and prospective memory

- Word retrieval and thought formulation for higher level complex verbal and written communication

- Complex information processing for listening and reading

- Executive functioning

- Reasoning, problem solving, and decision making

- Mathematical skills: computation and application

Following a case history review, client interview, client observation, careful scoring of tests, and interpretation of evaluation data, therapy may be recommended based on the individual's skill areas of impairment and intactness, as well as his or her motivation. It is at this point that the attention of the speech-language pathologist shifts to treatment. Developing specific, client-relevant treatment tasks for this higher level population requires knowledge of current literature, creativity, and meticulous planning. Treatment tasks may be utilized during individual sessions, in a small group setting, or in the community to integrate and apply relearned skills to realistic situations and environments.

Because individuals who have sustained mild-to-moderate TBIs may demonstrate great potential to return to independent living, school, and work, treatment may address underlying cognitive-language skills, as well as development of specific strategies related to independent living, return to work, and return to school. In addition, once the client has been reintegrated into an educational setting, therapy tasks may incorporate school course materials. If a job placement is secured, the clinician also may facilitate the client's success through strategy development, environmental modifications, and on-the-job assistance. To promote active therapy participation and maximal therapeutic benefit, it is important to involve the client in goal setting, task planning, and compensatory strategy development.

Sharing information with the client and his or her family is another role the speech-language pathologist must fulfill. The client and his or her family will require ongoing education and information regarding the injury, documented progress, developed compensatory strategies, and persisting cognitive-language concerns and how they affect the client's daily life. In addition, the client and his or her family will require support and direction from the speech-language pathologist over the course of treatment. Information conveyed to the client and his or her family may take the form of monthly reports, verbal updates, and telephone calls to keep the appropriate participants involved and active in the rehabilitation process. The family plays a vital role in assisting the client in transferring skills learned in therapy to the home, work, or school environment. Involving the family in each step of the rehabilitation process is crucial for maximizing the client's recovery and long-term skill maintenance.

INVOLVEMENT WITH THE ENTIRE REHABILITATION TEAM

Another responsibility of the speech-language pathologist working with individuals with mild-to-moderate TBI is to participate in the coordination of services among members of the rehabilitation team. In addition to the speech-language pathologist, the team may include a physiatrist or other medical specialist, insurance representative, case manager, psychologist, social worker, occupational therapist, physical therapist, recreational therapist, vocational counselor, or other professionals. Collaboration with each rehabilitation professional will ensure that the specific rehabilitation needs and goals of each client will be met during recovery. This interdisciplinary approach promotes functional, efficient, and cost-effective treatment services. Furthermore, a cooperative rapport creates increased understanding of each professional's respective role as a member of the rehabilitation team and helps to promote an improved outcome for the client. At times, differences in rehabilitation goals or approaches, inadequate communication, or territorial issues can hinder maximal team interaction.

Suggestions for being a "**team player**" include:

■ Don't set boundaries that limit you: increase your knowledge base.

■ Be flexible: look for connections between cognitive-language skills and daily living tasks, as these skills are required in many aspects of independent living.

■ Communicate often with other team members: ask questions, seek opinions and ideas, request support.

■ Remember that your overall goal is to foster the independent functioning of the client.

■ Remember that the client is a complex person with a variety of interrelated skill strengths, limitations, and needs.

COUNSELING AND EDUCATION OF CLIENTS AND FAMILY MEMBERS

Another responsibility within the realm of the clinician's numerous professional roles is to provide accurate information when educating and counseling individuals who have sustained a TBI and their family members. Fulfilling this therapeutic role assists in educating those involved in the family unit, validating many of the client's and family's concerns, building rapport to enhance ongoing discussion, and determining reasonable expectations to promote a favorable treatment outcome. Consistent communication among clinician, client, and family is critical to promote a professional comfort level for asking questions and sharing relevant and essential information. With the incorporation of managed care into the delivery of healthcare services, the number of treatment sessions may be limited in an effort to control the healthcare costs. "Capitation" limits either the number of therapy sessions authorized or the dollars available for continued treatment. The clinician must communicate to the client and family what needs to be accomplished in therapy within the authorized time frame. Additionally, the clinician has the responsibility of educating family members on useful compensatory strategies, cueing techniques, and home stimulation tasks for skill transfer and maintenance beyond the therapy environment. With this knowledge and the clinician's guidance, the client and his or her family will better understand how to maximize the treatment sessions available.

Providing counseling and enhancing others' knowledge and understanding of TBI may be an ongoing process. Many clinicians express discomfort with presenting themselves as "experts" when attempting to provide information regarding TBI or discussing specific facts when initially meeting with prospective referrals and their family members. To best prepare yourself for this role, it is important to consider the scope of your knowledge, your level of sensitivity, the amount of your clinical experience, and your willingness to defer to others when a question may be answered better by another professional. Disseminating accurate and useful information to others includes:

■ Utilizing clinical information learned from previous client experience

■ Collecting material and maintaining a review of recent journal articles

■ Reviewing book chapters, texts, and other current publications

■ Attending professional conferences relevant to this area of rehabilitation

Gaining further knowledge and experience will increase your level of understanding and expertise, which in turn will improve your ability to comfortably and accurately share information with your clients, their families, and your colleagues.

Counseling and educating clients and their families does not end after the initial meeting or evaluation process. Following the sharing of assessment results and the determination of treatment goals, the clinician continues to provide counseling and information throughout the duration of treatment. As will be presented in greater detail in the treatment section of this manual, clients who have experienced a mild-to-moderate TBI often are aware of their skill limitations and ask challenging questions pertaining to their deficits. This heightened awareness and anxiety prompts clients to develop a multitude of feelings and concerns, which the clinician must address as they arise during therapy sessions. Again, knowledge and experience are your best resources to answer questions directly, honestly, and professionally. Other suggestions to maintain a professional perspective include:

1. Supplement your discussions with documented facts and clinical observations within the scope of your experience and expertise.

2. If you do not know the answer to a question, say so and suggest another professional to consult (perhaps another team member who can better address the issue).

3. Do not let personal emotions or values interfere with your clinical judgment; respect your clients' personal goals and priorities.

4. Attempt to educate your client by providing written information such as journal articles, reference lists, and community resources to support your verbal comments and schedule a follow-up discussion, if necessary.

COORDINATION OF RETURN TO SCHOOL OR WORK WITH ADJUNCT EDUCATORS AND VOCATIONAL COUNSELORS

Returning to school or work is one of the primary goals of rehabilitation for adolescents and adults with mild-to-moderate TBI. When considering a client's potential to return to an academic or job setting, one of the responsibilities of the speech-language pathologist might be to assist in adding members to the treatment team. If a return to school or work is anticipated, contact should be made with the school counselor, teachers, or vocational counselor as early as possible in the rehabilitation process. Initially, the clinician serves as a resource, providing general information regarding TBI. When consulting with the teacher or vocational counselor regarding a specific client, the clinician outlines the client's skill strengths and limitations, useful compensatory strategies, and the unique needs of the client re-entering the educational setting or potential job environment. Sharing information with additional team members is an essential component in coordinating rehabilitation efforts, which may enable the client, rehabilitation specialists, educators, and counselors to work together efficiently and effectively.

Working Within the Educational and Vocational Systems

With the implementation of Public Law 101-476: Individuals with Disabilities Education Act, which includes TBI within special education laws (Americans with Disabilities Act, 1990), the transition of students from the rehabilitation setting back into the academic setting has improved during recent years. Advances have been made in the identification, placement, and educational programming for children, adolescents, and adults (up to age 26) with TBI. Issues such as how to classify students with TBI to meet their individual educational needs, and how to plan and monitor their academic programs remains a challenge for educators. Being aware of these issues and, more importantly, consistently targeting, monitoring, and modifying ways to meet the needs of these students are critical to their long-term educational success.

The Individual Educational Plan (IEP) process provides a format for the family, clinicians, and educators to discuss openly the types and frequency of support services that may be necessary to meet the student's needs. The speech-language pathologist is an integral component of this process, facilitating communication between the rehabilitation center and the school. This role is especially important to the client who is returning to college, because IEPs are not implemented at this level and professors are often unaware of students who may have learning difficulties as a result of a TBI. With these students, the speech-language pathologist may need to initiate communication with specific professors through a letter or verbal communication, outlining the individual student's cognitive-language limitations as they impact academic performance, the student's learning style, and any suggestions the professor may utilize to best instruct and help the student succeed (see Appendix 1-A). Additionally, the clinician may need to provide guidance regarding types of classes to take to maximize the client's strengths and success, as well as the number of classes to take to ensure a manageable schedule.

The inclusion of vocational counseling in a client's rehabilitation process consists of several components that should be addressed by a certified vocational specialist. These include:

- Participating in a thorough vocational assessment

- Receiving ongoing job counseling

- Exploring potential job placements

- Attempting supported job trials

- Utilizing job coaching services

- Receiving constructive feedback

- Participating in follow-up counseling

The speech-language pathologist's initial involvement focuses on communication with the vocational counselor during the evaluation period to provide an assessment of the client's work-related cognitive and communicative strengths and limitations. Providing a written outline of the client's capabilities is quite helpful. Additionally, the speech-language pathologist may serve as a consultant to the vocational counselor, who is attempting to locate jobs that the client can be both challenged by and successful at, given his or her capabilities. When considering the possibility of a job placement, the speech-language pathologist should suggest a trial therapy period for specific task training and development of strategies to enhance the client's chances of success. Further therapeutic intervention may consist of targeting skills that are required by potential job tasks, assisting in job site modification through compensatory strategy implementation or environmental changes, visiting the work site to fully understand the job demands and environment in which the client will be working, providing on-the-job assistance, training a job coach, educating the employer, advocating for the client's potential to be successful at a job (see Appendix 1-B), and providing additional therapeutic support to address remaining skill concerns. Clearly, ongoing communication with the vocational counselor and, in some cases, the employer is essential. Finally, supporting a recommendation of a gradual return to work through discussions with the client, provides a realistic and supportive transition from the treatment setting to the workplace environment.

Therapy Focus

When focusing treatment goals on returning to work or returning to school, a number of similar cognitive, psychosocial, and physical motor difficulties should be addressed by an interdisciplinary treatment team. The speech-language pathologist targets any of the following cognitive-language skill areas that may impact the client's successful reintegration:

- Complex attention and concentration

- Functional memory

- Word retrieval and thought formulation

- Complex information processing and integration

- Executive functioning (task planning, initiation, and completion)

- Reasoning and problem solving

- Reading and math

- Self-monitoring

- Development of compensatory strategies

Other skill areas addressed by the occupational and physical therapists may include:

- Sequencing and organization

- Balance and coordination

- Sensory processing and integration

- Physical endurance

- Vision and visual perception

- Gross and fine motor skills

Prior to a return to the work or school environments, therapy tasks target skill deficits to facilitate maximal skill improvement. Subsequently, instructing the client in various compensatory strategies for persisting skill limitations provides an opportunity to introduce methods of accomplishing tasks with greater ease and success. Strategies should be individualized and directed to specific academic courses or job tasks to enhance their usefulness and to engage the client in understanding their purpose and meaning, as well as the need to use them consistently. This approach is therapeutic and helpful for both the school and work settings. As the instructional process is often completed by trial and error to determine what works best for the client, promoting the client's self-monitoring and obtaining feedback regarding strategy effectiveness are essential. Client feedback and self-reports are useful in determining which strategies are the most effective and which need further development to promote lasting success for clients who are returning to work or school environments.

As described previously, the speech-language pathologist's role in the return-to-work or return-to-school transition process is varied and meaningful. The clinician plays a vital role, serving as a valuable resource and consultant to educators, vocational counselors, and employers to help bridge the gap between the controlled rehabilitation setting and the more realistic and quite challenging work and school environments to which individuals with mild-to-moderate TBI work so hard to return.

EDUCATION OF THE INSURER OR OTHER FUNDING SOURCE

An adjunct role and responsibility of clinicians, which few realize, may be to communicate regularly with the insurance company or other funding source. Communication may take the form of telephone calls, update letters, monthly reports, or team conferences. Although a nurse case manager is generally assigned to the client's case, the treating clinician is one of the most appropriate team members to provide the payor with an explanation of why treatment is reasonable, necessary, and beneficial. This explanation and education may be communicated through a telephone call, a letter accompanying the evaluation results, or a team meeting. Information provided should include:

- A concise description of the client's skill strengths and limitations

- A clear outline of the goals for treatment

■ The frequency and duration of therapy

■ The anticipated progress as it relates to the client's return to previous lifestyle activities such as work and school

Providing both the case manager and insurer with this detailed information enhances their understanding of the impact of the injury on the client's daily functioning and increases their willingness to authorize treatment. A useful method of securing initial authorization is to recommend a trial period of treatment for several months to best determine the client's motivation to improve and participate in therapy, and the benefit of treatment as indicated by the documented progress.

Following the initial authorization for treatment, thereby securing payment for services, continued communication and documentation is essential as therapy can often be extended for lengthy periods of time, depending on the client's response to treatment and ongoing rehabilitation needs. Monthly therapy progress reports (which generally accompany the billing statements) should be clear and concise, with documentation regarding:

■ The client's behavior

■ Progress toward treatment goals (including a description of several therapy tasks, objective measures, and a narrative summary)

■ Persisting skill limitations

■ Therapy concerns

■ Treatment goal modifications

■ Recommendations regarding therapy focus and treatment timeline

In addition, this is an opportune way to suggest the involvement of other team professionals, if necessary. As this format indicates, it is the responsibility of the therapist to educate the funding source regarding why the therapeutic services being provided are necessary and beneficial.

Unfortunately, many circumstances arise that create a disruption in this educational and cooperative process with the insurer, and therefore, authorization for treatment services may be compromised. More often than not, conflicts arise as a result of the specific benefit language used in the insurance policy. In many policies, particularly medical policies (e.g., Blue Cross/Blue Shield, HMOs, etc.), "speech and language" services are a covered benefit; however, "cognitive therapy" is not an authorized medical benefit. Generally, this is due to the misconception of the definition of "cognitive treatment" and the various professionals who use this terminology to describe any number of treatment methodologies. Try as we may to change how others view and interpret cognitive therapy, and promote a clearer understanding of what this treatment should entail, it is critical that we adhere to benefits that are covered by the policy language. As clinicians, we find it necessary to know the exact benefits covered prior to initiating services. This knowledge assists in accurate documentation and proper description of the treatment provided, utilizing language accepted, understood, and authorized by the funding source. For example, many "cognitive or thinking" skills, such as speed of information processing, working memory capacity, and thought formulation may also be considered "language" skills. Documenting these skills as language impairments and describing the impact they have on a client's daily functioning provides the insurer with more accurate information on which to make a determination regarding continued payment for treatment services. Finally, although correspondence with the funding source should be client-specific, detailing each client's unique rehabilitation needs, several examples of format and content have been provided for your reference when formulating your thoughts, educating the insurer, and ultimately advocating for your therapeutic services on behalf of your clients (see Appendixes 1-C and 1-D).

INVOLVEMENT IN LITIGATION AND PREPARATION FOR DEPOSITIONS AND TESTIMONY

Due to the increased difficulty in obtaining treatment services for individuals with mild-to-moderate TBI, an expanding responsibility of the speech-language pathologist is serving as an expert witness. Psychologist William Hambacher, Ph.D., (1995) defined an expert witness as "a person who, through education or training, has knowledge or skills not possessed by an ordinary person to help the trier of fact reach a conclusion" (p. 10) by clarifying issues and presenting scientific information. Expert witnesses testify in their areas of expertise, offering facts and opinions regarding their general knowledge of the scope of practice or specific information relative to a client who was or is being seen for treatment services. When working with people with TBI, it is not uncommon for speech-language pathologists to be asked to testify regarding their evaluation and treatment services. There are many reasons a speech-language pathologist may be called to testify through a deposition or court appearance regarding a client:

- Need for past, present, or future therapy

- Benefit from past, present, or future therapy

- Performance on objective measures

- Observed or reported functional limitations and their impact on vocational potential, learning potential, academic success, social interaction, and independent functioning

- Guardianship

- Need for compensatory items such as a computer, job coach, or home modifications

One of the paramount issues in personal injury cases, particularly with the mild-to-moderate TBI population, is the extent to which the deficits are found to be legitimate, as opposed to exaggerated, as a result of the alleged injury (Miller, 1992). Postconcussion syndrome refers to "the constellation of mental symptoms and functional impairments that patients with head injuries often suffered, even when there was no loss of consciousness or other sign of major neurological injury" (Miller, 1996, p. 6). In relation to this definition, exaggerated symptoms or fabricated deficits are often referred to as "malingering." Specifically, malingering has been defined in the *Diagnostic and Statistical Manual of Mental Disorders—Fourth Edition* (American Psychiatric Association, 1994) as "the intentional production of false or grossly exaggerated physical or psychological symptoms, motivated by external incentives such as avoiding military duty, avoiding work, obtaining financial compensation, evading criminal prosecution, or obtaining drugs" (p. 683). Due to the wide variety of possible complaints and symptoms, some medical professionals or claims representatives suggest to their clients that some of their complaints lack justification or that their symptoms appear to be out of proportion to the actual severity of the documented physical injury. When the clients are presented with this perspective, their progress in treatment may be significantly slowed or interrupted, particularly when further requests for treatment are disregarded or denied by the health-care payor. It is at this point that the process of litigation may begin and the clinician's role as an expert witness may be necessary for the client to obtain or continue needed therapy services. Although this may not be required for many clients, as a clinician treating this population you should be prepared for this challenging role.

Prior to meeting with professionals, an attorney will request, by a court-ordered sub-poena, *all* documentation regarding the referenced client. It is a sound idea to make note of whether the attorney in question is for the defendant or plaintiff and who represents your client, as you may be called to testify for either side. When asking the client (or guardian) to sign the release form to indicate authorization for information to be submit-ted, it is helpful to state who is requiring the records. Regardless of authorization, you *must* forward requested records, as a subpoena is sent by a court of law and the clinician or provider facility is obligated to comply. Requests for information typically require the following original documents:

■ Case history

■ Evaluation reports and test forms

■ Daily treatment documentation

■ Monthly progress reports

■ Reassessment information

■ Discharge reports

■ Billing statements

■ Any correspondence generated by the therapist or healthcare provider

Do not submit copies of information documented by other healthcare professionals or facilities, as this work was not generated from your facility.

Upon receipt of the information, either the defending or opposing attorney may sub-poena the treating therapist to provide expert testimony through a deposition or by appearing in court. Although most cases settle prior to an actual court date, a clinician should take seriously any request for a deposition or expert testimony as both are official procedures. Providing professional testimony may involve stating your opinion regarding: current literature, the case history, your clinical findings or those of other professionals, the impact of the client's limitations on his or her daily living, treatment goals, and doc-umented progress. The clinician must be fully prepared to answer any number of ques-tions presented by the attorneys representing both sides of the litigation case. Always keep in mind that your client may be subject to litigation at any time, which further sup-ports why treatment should always be clearly documented, justified, and functional. In addition, because psychosocial, physical, and vocational impairments may not be obvious under less demanding clinical conditions, it is imperative that, during therapy, the clini-cian, with the client's active involvement, simulate a variety of functional and realistic sit-uations that require simultaneous skill use (using more than one cognitive skill at the same time) to best determine the client's true abilities. This will enable you to provide objec-tive, accurate, and relevant information, as well as informed, realistic opinions regarding your client's actual capabilities.

Finally, it is important to note that it is *not* the role of the speech-language pathologist to diagnose the client with a TBI. When questioned, you should state that this is typically the responsibility of the physiatrist or neuropsychologist. Rather, the speech-language pathologist may diagnose and testify to the presence of speech, language and cognitive disturbances *resulting* from the TBI. Additionally, it is *not* the role of the speech-language pathologist to testify as to whether the client is malingering. When questioned, you may indicate that diagnosing malingering is within the realm of neuropsychologists, as their comprehensive test battery includes multiple, standardized assessments of malingering and TBI. Furthermore, it is acknowledged in the literature that neuropsychologists must consider a wide range of methodologies prior to offering a clinical opinion on a client's potential malingering (Nies & Sweet, 1994), thereby providing a more well-supported opinion.

When participating in any legal proceeding, several initial steps are essential to the clinician's thorough preparation. First, prepare and have available a current curriculum vita. Second, review current, applicable literature to cite, which is relevant to the case in question. Lastly, complete an in-depth review of the client file to answer questions pertaining to the following:

- Referral source

- Evaluation results

- Client abilities and limitations

- Treatment goals

- Therapy tasks

- Documented progress

- Treatment concerns

- Prognosis

- Impact of limitations on client's success at school, work, social relationships, and daily living skills

When providing testimony on these issues, attempt to preface your statements with phrases such as, "To the best of my knowledge," "In my opinion," and "Based on my experience," to avoid an attack on your expertise as compared to other professionals in your field of specialty. This may occur when two speech-language pathologists are asked to testify, most likely on opposing sides.

It is equally important to know what not to state during a deposition or witness testimony. Use caution when responding to questions beyond the scope of your clinical experience and expertise and avoid using absolute terms such as "always" and "never." When applicable, attempt to phrase statements in terms of possibilities and probabilities, rather than percentages (Hambacher, 1995). Be aware of leading questions, such as "Don't you agree with . . ." or "Aren't you saying . . .," and avoid appearing defensive. If you do not know the answer, say so. The more prepared and informed you are, the more accurate and consistent your testimony will be.

In conclusion, your role as the expert witness is to testify for the benefit of the court. Any opinion provided should be your best clinical assessment of the case.

APPENDIX 1-A

Sample Letter: Academic

January 21, 1997

Dr. LeeAnn Peterson
1212 Pinegrove Drive
Ann Arbor, MI 48324

RE: Jim Hughes

Dear Dr. Peterson,

I write to you on behalf of Jim who is a student in your Biology 101 class. I am a Speech-Language Pathologist working with Jim to assist with his limitations he incurred following a traumatic brain injury last year. Jim has successfully continued pursuit of his CAAD associate's degree with an overall G.P.A. of 3.4 and will be graduating after the summer term of this year, pending completion of his science and communications requirements.

To maximize his success with your course, I thought it might be helpful to inform you of his limitations and ways you may be assistive. While appearing to be very high functioning, Jim displays reduced functioning in the areas of auditory processing, recall of information, multi-step processing (listening and taking notes), reading interpretation, basic spelling, organization, speed of processing, and sustained and selective attention (maintaining attention especially in the presence of distractions). Given his area of concentration, extensive note-taking and memorization have not been required. In preparation for this class, therapy is providing Jim with techniques for effective note-taking and use of compensatory memory strategies for enhanced learning.

The outline you give is very helpful in providing Jim with organization and an indication of what information you will be presenting. He benefits from presentation of information in the order he expects, since he can easily become disorganized and distracted. Additionally, Jim benefits from your effort to write notes on the board. This ensures accurate processing and allows for time to take notes. I have encouraged Jim to audiotape the class as he benefits from repetition and a slowed presentation of verbal information. In addition, any visual representations of information presented during lecture will be helpful as Jim is a visual learner and his visual memory is superior to his auditory memory.

I have encouraged Jim to sit at the front of the class, especially while taking an exam so that he is not visually distracted. You will probably find he is unable to complete quizzes and tests in the allotted amount of time even when he knows the information well. This is due to his reduced speed of processing written information and slowed recall of details. If time becomes a critical factor, perhaps you would consider being flexible with time constraints. I have also encouraged Jim to visit you during your office hours to review any areas of concern or confusion. Any assistance you can provide Jim would be greatly appreciated. Flexibility from academic professionals is crucial to successful reintegration of people who have sustained traumatic brain injuries. Please call if you have any questions.

Sincerely,

Ruth O'Malley, M.A., CCC
Speech-Language Pathologist

APPENDIX 1-B
Sample Letter: Vocational

June 30, 1997

Dr. Jordon Stein
4397 Grand River
E. Lansing, MI 48856

RE: Barry Jackson

Dear Dr. Stein,

Barry began receiving speech-language therapy services at our facility. Since that time, Barry has consistently demonstrated skill improvement and has diligently completed therapy tasks with the focus of achieving full recovery. Barry's primary rehabilitation goal has been to return to his pre-injury work level and lifestyle.

Currently, Barry continues speech-language therapy services for approximately four hours per week. Treatment tasks focus on verbal expression and higher level speech skills (thought formulation, speed of information processing, and word retrieval). We anticipate a significant reduction in therapeutic services during the next month, as Barry continues to increase his job responsibilities and work hours from his current schedule. It is my professional opinion as a Speech-Language Pathologist, that Barry demonstrates the capability of returning to work on a full-time basis from this date on, at his previous job level. Any change from his previous job responsibilities should be made based on documented work performance. Barry should actively participate in all work projects, as he did prior to his injury, in order to reacquaint himself with job expectations. Barry has repeatedly demonstrated strong motivation to return to work, and he consistently displays motivation to respond to feedback and revise his work product accordingly. As discharge plans from rehabilitation are targeting mid-August, remaining therapy sessions from this date forward will be scheduled outside of work commitments. In all respects, Barry exhibits job readiness and the skill capabilities to return to full-time work, participating in staff and client interactions, and high-level job tasks. As a short-term feedback measure, it would be useful to have Barry's immediate Supervisor review his work, prior to its external distribution, for a period of three months.

Should there be any questions or concerns, please contact me.

Sincerely,

Maureen Wheatley, M.S., CCC
Speech-Language Pathologist

APPENDIX 1-C

Sample Letter: Reimbursement Dispute

January 21, 1997

Ms. Erica Wellstone
117 Commonwealth Ave
Boston, MA 01770

RE: Leah Lawrence

Dear Ms. Wellstone:

Thank you for taking the time to assist me in understanding the medical policy language that dictates the therapeutic services benefit for Leah. The following information should assist you in coordinating the policy benefits available with my treatment goals, which direct my therapy tasks.

As stated in my initial evaluation report, Leah was referred to our rehabilitation services in November 1996. It was her opinion, and that of her husband, that the speech services she was receiving were not meeting her rehabilitation needs. Subsequent to our initial meeting, it was necessary to review previous therapy reports and complete additional, essential speech-cognitive tasks to best identify specific skill limitations. A variety of skill impairments (such as information processing and retention, rapid word retrieval, reasoning, verbal expression) can occur in any combination, following a traumatic brain injury. In my initial evaluation report dated November 1996, I detailed many therapeutic tasks that assessed Leah's higher level speech skills, in order to outline any skill concerns that could limit her ability to complete job tasks independently and accurately. All therapy with Leah was provided by a certified speech-language pathologist. All evaluation and therapy tasks were related to her communication and more specifically, her ability to process information and verbally express her thoughts and ideas. Therefore, it is my understanding that the professional time spent in direct speech treatment should be reimbursed in full, under the benefit of Speech Therapy according to Leah's policy. Occupational and work-hardening tasks were not completed, as my professional licensing would not permit this type of therapy.

Currently, Leah continues receiving speech therapy services generally four hours per week. Treatment tasks focus on verbal expression and higher level speech skills (thought formulation, speed of processing, and word retrieval). We anticipate a significant reduction in therapeutic services within the next three months. Leah's personal rehabilitation goal is to make as full of a recovery as possible and a complete return to pre-injury work level and lifestyle. This is a realistic goal, in my opinion, as she has diligently completed therapy tasks to obtain nearly a full recovery. It is my professional opinion that Leah demonstrates the capability of returning to work on a full-time basis from this date on, at her previous job level. Our remaining therapy sessions will be scheduled outside of her work commitments. Your reconsideration of reimbursement action on this account would be greatly appreciated. Again, we thank you for your time and effort and await your response. I've included the outstanding November 1996 invoice and have added December and January statements for your review and payment. If you have any further questions or concerns, please do not hesitate to contact me at any time.

Sincerely,

Sam Watkins, M.S., CCC
Speech-Language Pathologist

APPENDIX 1-D

Sample Letter: Treatment Authorization

June 9, 1997

Mr. Robert Vance
23051 Heritage Park
Bloomington, IN 44625

RE: Ben Stock

Dear Mr. Vance:

Your claimant, Ben, was recently referred to our rehabilitation facility by his Case Manager and Neuropsychologist. It appears that Ben apparently sustained a "mild traumatic brain injury" during a motor vehicle accident on March 4, 1996, as indicated in the detailed neuropsychological evaluation forwarded with this correspondence, with Dr. Reeves' authorization. As Ben attempted to return to his demanding work environment, it became apparent to him that difficulties he was experiencing using his cognitive-language and thinking skills persisted. A complete cognitive-language evaluation was requested to assess Ben's current performance status as concerns exist regarding his decreased attention and concentration, reduced information processing, integration and recall, impaired task organization and completion, and reduced word retrieval. Therapeutic intervention would facilitate improvement in these cognitive skills and assist Ben in functioning more independently and successfully in his complex work environment.

To summarize, our preliminary assessment results indicate limitations in Ben's ability to process, integrate, and recall new information; sustain, alternate, and divide his attention; read and reason complex material; and efficiently retrieve words and organize his thoughts to clearly express his ideas. These reduced higher level cognitive skills interfere with his ability to complete complex job tasks independently. In my professional opinion, individual cognitive-language therapy on a short-term basis will facilitate improvement in these skill areas, as well as assist Ben in developing compensatory strategies. Following the completed assessment, I recommend individual cognitive therapy on a trial three-month basis to determine his skill improvement and potential for further progress. At that time, I will determine the need for continued therapeutic intervention. I will provide monthly progress notes detailing his treatment and documenting Ben's progress. Our facility will submit billing statements on a monthly basis for your review and reimbursement.

Please respond in writing regarding your authorization of this treatment plan. Should you have any questions or concerns, please contact our office at your convenience.

Sincerely,

Robin Bishop M.A., CCC
Speech-Language Pathologist

SOURCES OF ADDITIONAL INFORMATION

Counseling and Education

Bennett, T. (1992). Conceptualizing traumatic brain injuries. *The Journal of Head Injury, 3*(1), 21–28.

Kamhi, A. G. (1994). Toward a theory of clinical expertise in speech-language pathology. *Language, Speech and Hearing Services in Schools, 25,* 115–118.

Kay, T. (1986). *Minor head injury: An introduction for professionals* (pp. 1–12). Washington DC: Brain Injury Association, Inc.

Prigatano, G. P. (1995). Lectureship: The problem of lost normality after brain injury. *The Journal of Head Trauma Rehabilitation, 10*(3), 87–95.

Stahl, C. (1995). Undetected mild head injury can wreck lives. *Advance for Speech-Language Pathologists and Audiologists, 5*(18), 18.

Trace, R. (1995). Client-clinician-family relationships at heart of counseling in professions. *Advance for Speech-Language Pathologists and Audiologists, 5*(1), 12–13, 42.

Educational and Vocational Involvement

Goodall, P, Lawyer, H. L., & Wehman, P. (1994). Vocational rehabilitation and traumatic brain injury: A legislative and public policy perspective. *The Journal of Head Trauma Rehabilitation, 9*(2), 61–81.

Kay, T., & Silver, S. M. (1988). The contribution of the neuropsychological evaluation to the vocational rehabilitation of the head-injured adult. *The Journal of Head Trauma Rehabilitation, 3*(1), 65–76.

Kreutzer, J., Wehman, P., Morton, M., & Stonnington, H. (1988). Supported employment & compensatory strategies for enhancing vocational outcome following traumatic brain injury. *Brain Injury, 2*(3), 205–223.

Lamport-Hughes, N. (1995). Learning potential and other predictors of cognitive rehabilitation. *The Journal of Cognitive Rehabilitation, 13*(4), 16–21.

Parker, R. S. (1995). The distracting effects of pain, headaches, and hyper-arousal upon employment after "minor head injury." *The Journal of Cognitive Rehabilitation, 13*(3), 14–23.

Savage, R. C., & Wolcott, G. F. (1995). *An educator's manual: What educators need to know about students with brain injury.* Washington DC: Brain Injury Association, Inc.

Veach, R., & Taylor, M. (1989). Vocational placement of minor head injured survivors. *The Journal of Cognitive Rehabilitation, 7*(4), 14–16.

Wehman, P., Kreutzer, J., West, M., Morton, M., & Diambra, J. (1989). Cognitive impairment and remediation: Implications for employment following traumatic brain injury. *The Journal of Head Trauma Rehabilitation, 4*(3), 66–75.

Ylvisaker, M. (1995). Getting the word out: Helping students with TBI communicate more effectively. *TBI Challenge, 3*(2), 13–16.

Insurer and Funding Source

American Speech-Language-Hearing Association. (1994). *Managing managed care: A practical guide for audiologists and speech-language pathologists.* Rockville, MD: American Speech-Language-Hearing Association.

Litigation

Gelman, J. (1995). Preparing to take the stand as an expert witness. *Advance for Speech-Language Pathologists and Audiologists, 5*(48), 10–11, 24.

Lemmon, J., Keatley, M., Carnes, J., Acimovic, M., Josephs, E., & Purvis, J. (1995). Mild traumatic brain injury, psychological factors and the effects of the medico-legal system on recovery. *The Journal of Cognitive Rehabilitation, 13*(5), 4–11.

Miller, L. (1992). Back to the future: Legal, vocational, and quality-of-life issues in the long-term adjustment of the brain-injured patient. *The Journal of Cognitive Rehabilitation, 10*(5), 14–20.

Miller, L. (1996). Malingering in mild head injury and the post-concussion syndrome: Clinical, neuropsychological and forensic considerations. *The Journal of Cognitive Rehabilitation, 14*(4), 6–17.

CHAPTER 2

Assessment of Mild-to-Moderate Traumatic Brain Injury

NEUROPSYCHOLOGICAL EVALUATION AND ASSESSMENT CONSIDERATIONS

Prior to developing a cognitive-language evaluation protocol and determining specific assessment tasks, it is beneficial to review information documented by a neuropsychologist, if available. In general terms, neuropsychology is the study of brain-behavior relationships as applied to clinically presented problems and observations. An evaluation by a neuropsychologist can augment the speech-language pathologist's assessment, as the neuropsychological battery typically includes a wide variety of measures. When used with our target populations, the data obtained from a neuropsychological evaluation can document and describe the presence or absence of a TBI, as well as the nature and degree of disability. Information regarding baselines of behavior and areas of impairment and disability should be considered during the establishment of general rehabilitation recommendations and used for comparison when documenting progress.

Traditional neuropsychological assessment may include measurement of the following functions:

- **Mood and Behavior Changes:**
  may be due to actual brain damage or the client's emotional reaction to a change in level of functioning

- **Cognitive Abilities:**
  attention and concentration
  speed of information processing
  simultaneous processing

- **Language Abilities:**
  single word and sentence comprehension
  auditory discrimination
  expressive language

- **Memory and Learning:**
  verbal and visual memory
  immediate and delayed recall
  new learning

- **Intelligence: Verbal and Performance**
  general intelligence (IQ)
  verbal intelligence
  nonverbal intelligence (performance)

- **Executive Functioning:**
  setting goals
  planning steps
  executing goals
  evaluating performance

- **Academic and Achievement:**
  vocabulary
  reading
  spelling
  calculations

■ **Abstract Reasoning and Concept Formation:**
verbal and non-verbal problem solving and judgment

■ **Fine Motor Control and Speed:**
constructional ability
manual dexterity
motor strength and coordination

■ **Sensory and Perception:**
temporal orientation
visual perception
tactile sensation
visual organization

■ **Tests of Dissimulation:**
effort
motivation

■ **Personality Inventory and Psychosocial Factors**

Subsequent to the information obtained on the testing measures, the neuropsychologist can develop a framework for rehabilitation considerations by documenting results, describing observations, and explaining interpretations based on the client's behavior and performance during the lengthy testing sessions. The results of a comprehensive neuropsychological evaluation can be utilized for a variety of purposes including:

■ Identifying impact of trauma and emotional reaction

■ Determining interaction of physical complaints, cognitive symptoms, and behavioral and emotional factors

■ Recommending involvement of treatment team members

■ Directing rehabilitation efforts

■ Suggesting compensatory strategies

■ Dictating daily living and supervision needs

■ Assisting with educational planning

■ Guiding vocational counseling

■ Providing driving guidelines

As outlined above, the evaluation of a multitude of skill areas completed by the neuropsychologist can provide valuable information to the client, family members, and other treatment team members. Of particular interest to the speech-language pathologist is the assessment of the client's cognitive and language abilities, which provides an outline of strengths and limitations from which a more in-depth cognitive and language evaluation may continue. As traditional neuropsychological test batteries are not considered sensitive to the reduction in information processing capacity (Acimovic, Keatley, & Lemmon, 1993), or the extent of attention decrement in the mild TBI population, the speech-language pathologist must further assess these and other skill areas under a variety of conditions. In addition, standard neuropsychological assessments may lack environmental validity and reveal minimal information about an individual's daily functioning, particularly when the brain injury is mild (Lewkowicz & Whitton, 1995). Therefore, the neuro-psychological assessment protocol is insufficient by itself for validating a client's concerns in a variety of settings and for providing a framework for cognitive treatment. The speech-language pathologist can provide focused treatment goals by specifically addressing the client's concerns and skill breakdown through formal and informal testing as detailed in the following section.

Prior to Test Administration

Review of Records

In preparation for evaluating a new client, the first step is to read the available medical history, including previous evaluation and progress reports from other rehabilitation professionals, such as acute care therapists and the neuropsychologist. It is recommended that clinicians review information and generate a list of related questions, prior to meeting with the client. It is helpful if a family member attends the initial consultation session to clarify or supplement information. Particular attention should be given to the results of the neuropsychological examination, if available, to assist the speech-language pathologist in developing a preliminary protocol of possible cognitive-language skill areas to assess. If the neuropsychological examination report is not in the medical record, an effort should be made to obtain it or recommend that a neuropyschological evaluation be completed as soon as possible. In addition, the clinician should attempt to obtain any pertinent vocational or academic reports. Furthermore, the clinician should confirm the authorized length of time for the cognitive-language evaluation with his or her supervisor, the case manager, or the insurance representative. Four to 6 hours may be necessary for a thorough, functional assessment; however, future health care trends may limit the time allotted for evaluation. Although comprehensive testing may be ideal, due to time constraints, priority may need to be given to skill areas of paramount concern.

Client Interview

The next step of the evaluation process is to conduct a client interview. It is helpful to begin the discussion by describing the types of services available at your particular facility and how therapy has been assistive to others. This approach tends to create an atmosphere in which the client feels comfortable by initially listening and then discussing information that may be humiliating, frustrating, sad, or of a personal nature. These disclosures will provide the clinician with a better understanding of the client's needs. Furthermore, have the client confirm general biographical information, and discuss his or her medical history, educational background, vocational experience, and any previous therapy. Additionally, allow the client to describe how the injury occurred and what difficulties are being experienced. For more specific information, the clinician might ask "What types of difficulties are you experiencing at home, work, and school?" and request specific examples.

Some points to remember while listening to the client's explanation include:

1. Utilize the interview as an opportunity to observe the client's verbal expression skills, pragmatics, attention, awareness of skill limitations, and speed of information processing.

2. Display genuine concern for your client's frustrations, which will serve as a sign of understanding and empathy.

3. Document detailed notes for later comparison with test results and as a measure of functional improvement.

4. Consider the underlying reduced skills that may account for the client's problems and note appropriate tests to administer to assess these skills.

To gain further information, particularly if the client demonstrates difficulty with providing a thorough description of his or her concerns, you may wish to ask questions to elicit specific facts pertaining to home, job, or academic demands. (See Appendixes 2-A, 2-B, and 2-C for sample questionnaires.) Such questions, tailored for an individual client based on his or her case history, may elicit more useful information regarding changes in functioning, as well as goal outcomes for the future. Questions from each sample questionnaire may be combined depending on the client's stated concerns and desired treatment outcome.

Some points to remember while listening to the client's responses include:

1. Consider the underlying reduced skills that may account for the client's problems at home, work, or school, and note appropriate tests to administer to assess these skills.

2. Keep detailed notes for later comparison with test results and as a measure of functional improvement.

3. View the questionnaire discussion as another opportunity to observe verbal expression skills, pragmatics, attention, awareness of skill limitations, and speed of information processing.

4. Utilize acquired information for simulated testing situations and potential therapy tasks that are personally relevant to the client.

Developing Rapport

The last segment prior to actual test administration, which actually continues during therapy, is to begin to develop rapport with your client, with the goal of achieving a trusting, positive, friendly, and professional relationship. With this in mind, it is strongly recommended that the clinician who will be providing treatment also conduct the client interview and complete the assessment. To foster rapport, it is recommended that the clinician provide a basic explanation of mild or moderate TBI, briefly describing the physiology and neurology in understandable terms and linking it to the client's corresponding functional limitations (refer to the definition in the Preface to assist with explanation). Such information tends to validate and make sense of the changed abilities, behaviors, and emotions the client may be experiencing. Additionally, a discussion on how therapy may be assistive through compensation, relearning, and new learning can be useful. Finally, allow time for the client to ask any questions and relay additional personal concerns.

If possible, arrange for the client to meet other clients with similar limitations. This is particularly useful for individuals with mild TBI as they are often misunderstood and many feel isolated. Encourage the other clients to explain their therapy and how it helped them, elaborating on their personal skill concerns, how they were functioning when beginning therapy, and what improvements they have made. In addition, allow the new client to ask any questions as this discussion format can be quite informative. Clients who are provided with this opportunity often report feeling they could truly relate to someone who had a similar experience. This tends to relieve and empower the new client, as well as validate his or her situation and feelings. It also provides current or former clients the opportunity to feel helpful to someone else.

Finally, discuss the general test procedure and time schedule. Completion of the evaluation on two different days is preferred to avoid fatigue. Subsequent to the client interview and initial testing, modifications may need to be made to the preliminary protocol. Explain to the client that test results will be provided in verbal and written reports that integrate all of the information, and that a meeting will be scheduled in the near future to review and explain the assessment conclusions and recommendations. This meeting and sharing of the evaluation results is an essential, yet sometimes deleted, component to the assessment protocol. It provides the client and family with an understanding of how a mild-to-moderate TBI can affect cognitive and daily living skills and the impact it can have on an individual's functioning at home, work, or school. It also provides an opportunity for additional questions and information-sharing, as well as the time to explain the team recommendations and next step in rehabilitation.

Once completed, this segment of the evaluation will have provided a clear idea of an individualized test protocol based on the information obtained during the interview. This information provides a more narrowly defined and targeted set of skills to assess and should assist the clinician in creating a personally relevant evaluation for each client given his or her preinjury functioning and treatment goals.

THE IMPORTANCE OF AN INTEGRATED ASSESSMENT

Upon completion of initial information-gathering through the client interview and review of available medical records and previous treatment reports, the evaluation process by the speech-language pathologist begins to assess the client's skill strengths and limitations as they relate to communicative and cognitive abilities, daily functioning, and work or school performance. Depoy's (1992) review of recent research and literature reveals an ongoing dilemma between the selection, use, and value of standardized and nonstandardized testing of individuals with mild-to-moderate TBI. This section will address this issue to assist the speech-language pathologist in determining the best possible approach for assessing each client.

Standardized, formal evaluation tools utilize specific procedures for test administration, which allow comparison of results with normative data. Quantitative, objective results indicate if a significant difference exists between the client's score and the standardized performance by others within a normed population. However, a client with mild-to-moderate TBI may perform "within normal limits" on all objective test measures, despite experiencing subtle yet "real" limitations that significantly impact daily functioning. For example, a client may demonstrate "normal" memory skills on a standardized test; however, if environmental distractors are introduced into the background while the client is attempting to encode the information, he or she may demonstrate inaccurate information retrieval due to improper encoding.

The ability to inhibit attention to distractions, so often required for success in work or school, is not typically incorporated into a standardized testing situation. Therein lies the major difficulty in utilizing current standardized evaluation protocols with this population: reduced sensitivity of testing does not clearly define areas of subtle skill breakdown. *The goal of a comprehensive evaluation is to clearly identify skill limitations that con-*

tribute to a client's reduced functioning capacity, as it is these higher level clients who demonstrate the best potential to return to work, home, and school responsibilities. There-fore, it is in the client's best interest for the clinician to utilize specific test modifications to discover subtle areas of skill breakdown to assist with appropriate treatment planning. For example, attention deficits and reduced speed of processing are generally displayed when time constraints are enforced or distractions are integrated into the testing envi-ronment. The clinician must evaluate the individual during similar conditions through modified formal and informal tests, simulated tasks, and assessment situations. Addi-tionally, use of a single complete evaluation battery may not be appropriate. Therefore, careful selection of specific subtests based on information provided (reports, discussion) will more accurately indicate the client's current skills while identifying areas of weak-ness. The evaluating clinician must place a high value on the responses provided by the client during the initial interview stage (see Appendixes 2-A, 2B, and 2C), as these re-sponses will guide the selection of assessment materials. Clinical observations of behav-ior and interpretation of information provided by the client, during both the interview and testing, will enable the clinician to identify possible underlying skill concerns necessary for adapting the evaluation protocol.

Because formal assessment procedures have limited use in the mild-to-moderate TBI population when used alone, informal measures are necessary to offer a complete pattern of the client's strengths and limitations. Current research on the assessment preferences of practicing speech-language pathologists by Frank and Barrineau (1996) indicates that a thorough assessment should incorporate results from both formal and informal evaluation protocols. Thus, one may select a specific standardized test to use informally through pro-cedure modifications, such as adding noise distractors in the background during a formal test. Furthermore, the clinician may create individualized testing situations that simulate personally relevant work, home, or school tasks. For example, a person previously employed as an executive assistant may be required to collate reports and answer telephone calls dur-ing an informal testing situation to assess complex attention, information processing speed and accuracy, and the use of several skills simultaneously. Utilizing simulated situations allows for observational methods of gathering functional and qualitative information. In conjunction with formal test results, these approaches will yield a complete view of the client's specific areas of strength and limitation, as well as provide direction and focus for appropriate treatment goals and therapy tasks.

In summary, a comprehensive evaluation battery, consisting of both formal and in-formal measures, will provide clinicians with useful information with which to structure an appropriate treatment plan that addresses unique treatment needs for the client's optimum benefit. This integrated approach, using the client interview, clinical observa-tion, and formal and informal testing provides essential data for clinical management. To obtain results that document the range of an individual's impairments and disabilities, the clinician should utilize:

1. Formal (standardized) evaluation tests

2. Informal measures such as modified test procedures and nonstandardized tasks

3. Clinical observations

4. Simulated situations

In addition, the clinician should carefully observe and interpret the full range of behav-iors and scores to clarify specific client concerns. This methodology will provide the clin-ician with the most realistic illustration of the client's current functioning capacity.

TEST ADMINISTRATION

The authors' preferences for testing individuals with mild-to-moderate TBI are described in this section. Our protocol includes formal tests; however, because many of these tests are insensitive to the subtle deficits of the person with mild TBI, we recommend modified formal and informal tests, clinical observations, and simulated situations relevant to a specific client's work, school, and lifestyle. We have found that this more flexible protocol usefully and efficiently documents the client's strengths and limitations to establish realistic goals of treatment. For example, we recommend utilization of an observation checklist to be completed throughout the evaluation to assist in documentation of clinical observations not measured by formal testing. It is important to document such behaviors as they may indicate the reason for functional difficulty in clients who perform well on standardized tests. Additionally, they provide information on how deficits may manifest themselves in work, home, and school (see Appendix 2-D). As evaluation time authorized by the insurer may not allow for extended assessment tasks, clinical judgment must be used to determine what skill areas should be addressed in depth through simulated situations prepared in advance. Subsequently, functional therapy tasks may then be planned and implemented to maximize the client's potential to return as close as possible to preinjury functioning. In the following section, the information is organized according to each skill area to be assessed.

COMPLEX ATTENTION
(Sustained, Selective, Alternating, Divided)

PARAMETERS TO EVALUATE:

1. Ability to sustain attention

2. Ability to inhibit internal and external distractions

3. Ability to shift focus of attention with ease

4. Ability to simultaneously focus attention on more than one stimulus

STANDARDIZED TESTS:

Test of Everyday Attention (TEA) (Robertson, Ward, Ridgeway, & Nimmo-Smith, 1994)
Paced Auditory Serial Addition Test (PASAT) (Gronwall, 1977)

MODIFIED TESTS:

Speed and Capacity of Language Processing (SCOLP) (Baddeley, Emslie, & Nimmo-Smith, 1992). Administer with and without talk radio in background and compare performance

CLINICAL OBSERVATIONS:

Observation of attentional skills during initial interview and other testing situations (utilize Appendix 2-D).

SIMULATED SITUATIONS:

Simulate a job, school, or home task the client reports as difficult to determine if it is reduced attention that may be interfering.

Examples:

■ Have the client talk on the telephone and obtain information while you talk in the background with another person.

■ Leave the therapy room door open and have the client verbally present information to you while other staff and clients walk by the room.

INTEGRATION OF OTHER TEST RESULTS:

Consider the impact of reported physical complaints such as headaches, pain, and fatigue on attention.

MEMORY SKILLS

(New Learning and Prospective Memory)

PARAMETERS TO EVALUATE:

1. Amount of information encoded accurately across modalities

2. Amount of information retained accurately

3. Amount of information retrieved accurately

4. Length of time for which information is retained

5. Speed of information presented without affecting memory encoding, storage, and retrieval

STANDARDIZED TESTS:

California Verbal Learning Test (CVLT) (Delis, Kramer, Kaplan, & Ober, 1987)

Scales of Cognitive Ability for Traumatic Brain Injury (SCATBI)—Recall Subtest (Adamovich & Henderson, 1992)

Learning Efficiency Test II (LET-II) (Webster, 1992)

Associate Learning Subtest of the *Wechsler Memory Scale—3* (Wechsler, 1997)

Prospective Memory Screening (PROMS) (Sohlberg & Mateer, 1989)

CLINICAL OBSERVATIONS:

Observation of memory skills during initial interview and other testing situations (utilize Appendix 2-D).

SIMULATED SITUATIONS:

Simulate a job, school, or home task the client reports as difficult to determine if reduced memory skills may be interfering.

Examples:

■ Instruct the client to obtain items from various rooms in the facility according to your verbal instructions.

■ Instruct the client to send you a note with specific requested information after the evaluation.

INTEGRATION OF OTHER TEST RESULTS:

Consider the impact of reduced attention and organization on memory skills by reviewing test performance within these skill areas.

VERBAL COMMUNICATION SKILLS
(Word Retrieval, Thought Formulation, Expression)

PARAMETERS TO EVALUATE:

1. Speed and ease of retrieving words and thoughts

2. Thought organization

3. Verbosity

4. Tangentiality

5. Maintaining train of thought and level of distractibility

6. Reasoning and coherent train of thought

7. Fluency

STANDARDIZED TESTS:

The Adolescent Word Test (Zachman, Barrett, Huisingh, Orman, & Blagden, 1989)
Scales of Cognitive Ability for Traumatic Brain Injury (SCATBI)—Word Generation of the Recall
     Subtest (Adamovich & Henderson, 1992)

NONSTANDARDIZED TASKS:

Evaluation of verbal communication skills while discussing any of the following:

■ job tasks

■ school assignments

■ daily home tasks

■ current events

■ pros/cons of an issue

CLINICAL OBSERVATIONS:

Observation of verbal communication skills during initial interview and other testing
situations (utilize Appendix 2-D).

SIMULATED SITUATIONS:

Simulate a job, school, or home task the client reports as difficult to determine if verbal communication skills are interfering.

Example:

■ Have the client (and clinician) review a personally-relevant article (one to three
pages) and have the client verbally outline main points and briefly summarize
information in a succinct manner.

INTEGRATION OF OTHER TEST RESULTS:

Consider the impact of reduced attention, memory, reasoning, and organization on
verbal communication when reviewing test performance in those skill areas.

WRITTEN COMMUNICATION SKILLS

(Word Retrieval, Thought Formulation, Expression)

PARAMETERS TO EVALUATE:

1. Speed and ease of retrieving words and thoughts
2. Sentence and paragraph organization
3. Tangentiality
4. Maintaining train of thought and level of distractibility
5. Reasoning and coherent train of thought, thought clarity
6. Ability to integrate thoughts comprehensively, yet concisely

STANDARDIZED TESTS:

Scholastic Abilities Test for Adults (SATA) (Bryant, Patton, & Dunn, 1991)

MODIFIED TESTS AND NONSTANDARDIZED TASKS:

To increase difficulty of the *Scholastic Abilities Test for Adults* (SATA) (Bryant, Patton, & Dunn, 1991), provide a more complex picture about which to write.

Use the *General Educational Development* (GED) practice book (Research and Education Association, 1992) composition section to test paragraph and essay writing.

Have the client write about any of the following:

■ pros/cons of an issue

■ job tasks

■ school assignments

■ daily home tasks

■ current events

CLINICAL OBSERVATIONS:

Discuss in detail any writing concerns the client has reported and consider possible underlying skills that may contribute to described limitations.

SIMULATED SITUATIONS:

Simulate a job, school, or home task the client reports as difficult to determine if written expression skills are interfering.

Examples:

■ Have the client write a typical work-related sample (explaining a job policy or procedure) with noise in the background or periodic verbal interruptions.

■ Have the client produce a writing sample by formulating a letter of complaint to a company regarding a defective product and how the issue should be resolved to his or her satisfaction.

INTEGRATION OF OTHER TEST RESULTS:

Consider the impact of reduced attention, memory, reasoning, and organization on written communication by reviewing test performance within these skill areas.

VERBAL INFORMATION PROCESSING SKILLS
(Listening and Auditory Processing)

PARAMETERS TO EVALUATE:

1. Speed of processing

2. Length of information able to process accurately

3. Complexity of information able to process accurately and easily

4. Comprehension

5. Retention

6. Application and utilization

STANDARDIZED TESTS:

Clinical Evaluation of Language Functions (CELF)—Ambiguities Subtest (Semel-Mitz & Wiig, 1982)

Clinical Evaluation of Language Functions (CELF)—Oral Directions Subtest (Semel-Mitz & Wiig, 1982)

Detroit Tests of Learning Aptitude—2 (DTLA-2)—Following Directions Subtest (Hammill, 1985)

Scales of Cognitive Ability for Traumatic Brain Injury (SCATBI)—Recall Subtest (Adamovich & Henderson, 1992)

NONSTANDARDIZED TASKS:

Listen to talk radio segment and have client verbally summarize information.

CLINICAL OBSERVATIONS:

Observation of listening skills during initial interview and other testing situations (utilize Appendix 2-D).

SIMULATED SITUATIONS:

Simulate a job, school, or home task the client reports as difficult to determine if verbal information processing skills are interfering.

Examples:

■ Present several work-related directions to follow, with and without people talking in the background, varying the number of directions provided at one time.

■ Explain topical information from a magazine or newspaper and have the client write down key words to assist with accurately answering questions posed by the clinician.

INTEGRATION OF OTHER TEST RESULTS:

Consider the impact of reduced attention, speed of processing, language comprehension, memory, or reasoning on verbal information processing skills by reviewing test performance within those skill areas.

WRITTEN INFORMATION PROCESSING SKILLS
(Reading Comprehension and Retention)

PARAMETERS TO EVALUATE:

1. Speed of processing

2. Length of information able to process accurately

3. Complexity of information able to process accurately and easily

4. Comprehension

5. Retention

6. Application and utilization

STANDARDIZED TESTS:

Gray Oral Reading Tests—Revised (GORT–R) (Wiederholt & Bryant, 1986)
Speed and Capacity of Language Processing (SCOLP) (Baddeley, Emslie, & Nimmo-Smith, 1992)
Scholastic Abilities Test for Adults (SATA)—Vocabulary Subtest (Bryant, Patton, & Dunn, 1991)
Scholastic Abilities Test for Adults (SATA)—Comprehension Subtest (Bryant, Patton, & Dunn, 1991)

MODIFIED TESTS:

Speed and Capacity of Language Processing (SCOLP) (Baddeley, Emslie, & Nimmo-Smith, 1992) with talk radio in background (use two of the four different versions provided)
Gray Oral Reading Tests—Revised (GORT-R) (Wiederholt & Bryant, 1986) with and without reference to paragraphs when responding to questions (use the two different versions provided)

CLINICAL OBSERVATIONS:

Note any frustration or delays in processing during reading testing.

SIMULATED SITUATIONS:

Simulate a job, school, or home task the client reports as difficult to determine if reading skills are interfering.

Examples:

■ Have the client review informative sources such as popular news magazine articles (8 to 10 paragraphs in length) and write a summary of the information presented. The client should be permitted to refer back to information read to limit the interference of reduced memory skills.

■ If aware of the client's academic or vocational focus, attempt to utilize related reading materials.

INTEGRATION OF OTHER TEST RESULTS:

Consider the impact of reduced attention, speed of processing, language comprehension, memory, and reasoning on written information processing skills by reviewing test performance in those skill areas.

EXECUTIVE FUNCTIONING SKILLS

(Planning, Initiating, Self-Monitoring)

PARAMETERS TO EVALUATE:

1. Goal selection
2. Planning and sequencing
3. Initiation
4. Task completion
5. Time sense
6. Awareness of change in functioning
7. Self-monitoring

STANDARDIZED TESTS:

Profile of Executive Control System (PRO-EX) (Broswell et al., 1992)

NONSTANDARDIZED TASKS:

Note if client completes the Client Response to Assessment form (see Appendix 2-E), which provides information on the client's initiation, self-monitoring, and task completion skills.

CLINICAL OBSERVATIONS:

Discuss in detail any executive functioning problems as reported by the client (e.g., "I can't seem to complete tasks," "I don't ever seem organized.")

SIMULATED SITUATIONS:

Simulate a job, school, or home task the client reports as difficult to determine if executive functioning skills are interfering.

Examples:

■ Present the client with a disorganized file cabinet and request assistance with organizing it. (Evaluates planning, organization, and task completion skills)

■ Request the client to devise a detailed schedule to successfully complete job or school demands for one week. (Evaluates goal-setting, planning, organization, and time sense)

INTEGRATION OF OTHER TEST RESULTS:

Consider the impact of reduced attention, memory, and organization on executive functioning skills by reviewing test performance in these skill areas.

REASONING SKILLS

(Concrete, Abstract, Decision Making, Problem Solving)

PARAMETERS TO EVALUATE:

1. Ability to think abstractly

2. Ability to solve complex problems

3. Ability to make sound decisions

4. Verbal reasoning during discussions

5. Ability to retain and integrate multiple factors while reasoning

STANDARDIZED TESTS:

Scales of Cognitive Ability for Traumatic Brain Injury (SCATBI)—Reasoning and Quantitative Reasoning Subtest (Adamovich & Henderson, 1992)

Scholastic Abilities Test for Adults (SATA)—Verbal, Nonverbal, and Reasoning Subtests (Bryant, Patton, & Dunn, 1991)

NONSTANDARDIZED TASKS:

Present controversial topic and have the client provide an opinion and defense position (to increase level of difficulty, complete task with background distractions)

Read complex word problems and have the client solve computations in a noisy environment (e.g. talk radio, door open, others in background).

CLINICAL OBSERVATIONS:

Observation of reasoning skills during initial interview and other testing situations (utilize the Observation Checklist in Appendix 2-D).

Discuss in detail any reasoning, problem-solving, and decision-making problems the client has reported.

SIMULATED SITUATIONS:

Simulate a job, school, or home task the client reports as difficult to determine if reasoning, problem-solving, or decision-making skills are interfering.

INTEGRATION OF OTHER TEST RESULTS:

Consider the impact of reduced attention, memory, and language processing on reasoning skills by reviewing test performance in these skill areas.

MATHEMATICAL SKILLS

PARAMETERS TO EVALUATE:

1. Computation
2. Application

STANDARDIZED TESTS:

Scholastic Abilities Test for Adults (SATA)—Math Computation Subtest and Math Application Subtest (Bryant, Patton, & Dunn, 1991)

NONSTANDARDIZED TASKS:

Functional math story problems regarding time and money solved in the presence of background distractions

Provide practice problems from the *General Educational Development* (GED) book (Research and Education Association, 1992) or other math practice workbooks.

CLINICAL OBSERVATIONS:

Discuss in detail any reasoning, problem-solving, and decision-making problems the client has reported in relation to mathematical skills such as grocery shopping, bill paying, and banking.

SIMULATED SITUATIONS:

Simulate a job, school, or home task the client reports as difficult to determine if math skills are interfering.

INTEGRATION OF OTHER TEST RESULTS:

Consider the impact of reduced attention, self-monitoring, memory, organization, and reasoning on math skills by reviewing test performance in these skill areas.

PREPARING THE COGNITIVE-LANGUAGE EVALUATION REPORT

A meaningful interpretation and a comprehensive report of the assessment results require the clinician to analyze and integrate all of the information learned from the client interview, standardized testing measures, nonstandardized tasks, clinical observations, and simulated task situations.

Analyzing Test Scores

Test results may be reported in various formats depending on the testing measure and type of information desired. Standardized assessment measures typically provide a standard score or percentile rank as compared to a normative population. Modified tests, nonstandardized tasks, and simulated situations may be described comparatively or qualitatively. For instance, when administering the same formal test with and without talk radio in the background as a distraction, the clinician should report the percentage of correct responses in each situation. Additionally, it is helpful to use descriptive terms that relate to more functional tasks such as "Harold demonstrated the ability to follow two-step commands presented in a quiet environment and single-step commands with distractions in the background. This may explain why he is experiencing difficulty following lengthy verbal directions at home and work." Lastly, information learned during the client interview and through observation during testing should supplement the standardized test scores. This method results in a more holistic and realistic interpretation of the client's difficulties and relates the objective score to the real-life skill limitations the client is reportedly experiencing.

To illustrate, a person may score within the normal range on a memory test as indicated by the standard score; however, he or she may be mentally fatigued following the testing and unable to adequately function the remainder of the day. This may indicate either the excessive level of energy required to perform successfully on a single mental task or sensory overload as a result of task demands. Clearly, such information is important when discussing a client's limitations and how they may be interfering with his or her successful return to home activities, work responsibilities, or school demands. Additionally, such information assists in guiding treatment goals and approaches to remediation. Such types of qualitative indicators, including frustration tolerance, level of effort, physical discomfort, sensory overload, and fatigue, may be observed by the clinician or reported by the client during the evaluation.

As an alternative, the clinician may provide the client with a brief questionnaire to complete at home for more detailed information regarding how the client felt physically and mentally following the testing (see Appendix 2-E: Client Response to Assessment). Thus, for any given test, the clinician must look beyond the test score, because an interpretation based strictly on a number score may be misleading, unfair to the client, and inaccurate in reflecting the nature of the skill deficits.

To further support the importance of test interpretation beyond the score, consider the situation where a client achieves a normal standard score on an auditory processing test, but, when audible distractions are introduced in the background (to more closely simulate the natural work environment), his or her performance is significantly compromised. A strict interpretation of the standardized score would not indicate the need for therapy for this client who may then return to work only to face repeated failures. In treatment, the client can practice and relearn efficient skill use through creative therapy tasks. Thus, a thorough assessment and interpretation with equal priority given to the client interview, standardized tests, nonstandardized tasks, clinical observations, and simulated situations are essential to obtain a true picture of the deficits of individuals with mild-to-moderate TBI.

Interpreting Supplemental Information

When testing has been completed and the tests have been scored, it is necessary to review all of the other qualitative information obtained to gain a full understanding of the client's functional limitations and to formulate clinical opinions. The following suggestions are offered to assist in this task:

1. Link test performance with concerns reported by the client during the client interview to best judge what skill impairments may be attributed to the cognitive and language difficulties experienced.

2. Be extremely observant during the client interview, discussion, and all testing situations, with special attention given to the following:
    a. fatigue during and after testing
    b. speed of individual test completion
    c. level of frustration
    d. sources of frustration
    e. stimulus overload and the need for timed breaks
    f. evidence of cognitive struggling
    g. requests for repetition
    h. ability to consistently self-monitor and self-correct
    i. effect of time pressure on performance
    j. performance following introduction of distractions (See Appendix 2-D: Observation Checklist to assist with recording information during testing).

3. Review test responses and document the number and types of errors. It is not uncommon for individuals with mild-to-moderate TBI to score incorrectly on some easier questions and score correctly on more difficult questions. This may be explained by *cerebral inefficiency*, which describes periodic, brief lapses in the brain's attentive, efficient functioning.

4. Compare and contrast different results from tests that measure similar cognitive-language skills by reporting quantitative and qualitative information.

5. Compare test performance in each of the language modalities of reading, writing, listening, and speaking to better understand the client's strengths and limitations.

Sharing Assessment Results

Typically, a written report is prepared and discussed with the client and treatment team at a family meeting. Written reports may be presented in a brief objective format or a more lengthy narrative format. We recommend a narrative format for the mild-to-moderate TBI population as this allows for discussion and integration of the supplemental qualitative and nonstandardized information. (See the sample evaluation sections provided in Appendix 2-F). It is useful to separate test results by skill area, incorporating all tests and observations with a final statement about that specific skill area regarding degree of impairment. A final summary paragraph should state all skill strengths and limitations (see sample summary in Appendix 2-F). Following this discussion, it is necessary to outline recommendations and indicate if treatment is warranted. If therapy would be beneficial, initial therapy goals and objectives, as well as recommendations for therapy frequency and duration, should be included. We find it appropriate to recommend therapy on a trial basis for an initial period of time, such as 3 months, to determine benefit to the client and to document progress in therapy. Subsequently, additional recommendations for further treatment may be made. The following suggestions are provided for verbal or written presentation of evaluation results:

■ Discuss strengths first to set a positive tone

■ Discuss limitations clearly, sensitively, and diplomatically

■ Relate test performance to specific cognitive-language problems and frustrations reported by the client

■ Relate skill strengths and limitations to the potential to return to work or school (see Job Implications in Appendix 2-G).

■ Respond to questions about prognosis honestly, realistically, and with as much optimism as is appropriate

■ Briefly explain how therapy may be helpful, focusing on skill improvement through practice and development of useful compensatory strategies.

■ Provide an opportunity for the client or family member to ask any further questions, as this is an opportune time for sharing information and explaining how a mild-to-moderate TBI can impact an individual's daily functioning in a variety of situations.

APPENDIX 2-A
Client Interview—Home Questionnaire

Select from these questions to elicit more specific information during the client interview regarding the level of functioning in the home environment.

Describe a typical day relative to your home responsibilities and schedule.

Describe your home environment. Are you easily distracted?

What do you find most challenging or frustrating about home?

How soon do you fatigue (e.g., after ___ hours)?

Describe the general amount (approximate minutes or hours) of time each day you rely on:

- reading
- writing
- speaking
- listening

How would you rate the strength of each skill when comparing them to each other? What skills seem to be your strongest and what are your weakest?

In terms of time and time management, describe demands on your time such as deadlines, speed of task completion, and multiple assignments. What is difficult for you?

Describe your organizational style and memory system. What strategies do you use to accomplish tasks?

Describe any other strategies or people you rely on to assist you in completing daily tasks and handling household and family demands.

In your opinion, what type of therapeutic assistance do you need?

APPENDIX 2-B
Client Interview—Work Questionnaire

Select from these questions to elicit more specific information during the client interview regarding the level of functioning in the work environment.

Describe a typical day relative to your job responsibilities, sample work tasks, and your schedule.

Describe your overall concerns regarding your thinking skills and potential to work in your field of interest.

What do you find most challenging or frustrating about work?

Describe your work environment:

- quiet or interactive
- independent work or team effort
- correspondence: telephone, in person, letter writing

Are you easily distracted?

How soon do you fatigue (e.g., after ___ hours)?

What specific skills do you use to complete your job tasks?

Which skills are lacking? How does this impact your job performance?

Describe the general amount (approximate minutes or hours) of time each day you rely on:

- reading
- writing

- ■ speaking

- ■ listening

How would you rate the strength of each skill when comparing them to each other? What skills seem to be your strongest and what are your weakest?

In terms of time and time management, describe demands on your time such as deadlines, speed of task completion, and multiple assignments. What is difficult for you?

Describe your organizational style and memory system. What strategies do you use to accomplish tasks?

Describe any other strategies or people you rely on to assist you in completing daily tasks and handling work assignments.

What are your educational goals relative to a possible future change in job choice?

In your opinion, what type of therapeutic assistance do you need?

APPENDIX 2-C
Client Interview—School Questionnaire

Select from these questions to elicit more specific information during the client interview regarding the level of functioning in the school environment.

What recent coursework have you completed and what were your grades?

Describe your overall concerns regarding your learning skills and potential to succeed in school.

Are there additional courses you are planning to take?

What do you find easiest about school?

What do you find most challenging or frustrating about school?

Describe your school environment:

Are you easily distracted?

How soon do you fatigue (e.g., after ___ hours)?

Describe the general amount of time each day you rely on:

■ reading

■ writing

- speaking

- listening

How would you rate the strength of each skill when comparing them to each other? What skills seem to be your strongest and what are your weakest?

In terms of time and time management, describe demands on your time such as deadlines, speed of task completion, and multiple assignments. What is difficult for you?

Describe your organizational style and memory system. What strategies do you use to accomplish academic assignments?

Describe any other strategies or people you rely on to assist you in completing daily tasks and handling academic demands.

What are your educational goals relative to a future job?

In your opinion, what type of therapeutic assistance do you need?

APPENDIX 2-D
Observation Checklist

Client _____

Date: _____

Factors to Observe and Document:

☐ **Displays overload**
    ☐ asks you to wait before presenting next stimulus item
    ☐ requests repetition
        ☐ average number of requests
    ☐ requests a break
        ☐ number of requests
        ☐ average number of breaks
    ☐ demonstrates confusion (e.g., does not appear to understand test instructions)

Additional Notes:

☐ **Displays fatigue**
    ☐ verbally reports fatigue and difficulty concentrating
    ☐ physically demonstrates fatigue (eye closing, facial grimacing, head lowering)

Additional Notes:

☐ **Demonstrates frustration**
    ☐ vents frustration verbally
    ☐ vents frustration physically
    ☐ refuses further participation in testing
    ☐ regains control independently
    ☐ regains control with clinician's encouragement
    ☐ resumes testing after a break

Additional Notes:

☐ **Speed of response**
    ☐ slow or delayed (struggling)
    ☐ adequate for testing purposes
    ☐ fast (impulsive)

Additional Notes:

☐ **Ability to self-correct**
- ☐ consistent and independent
- ☐ inconsistent
- ☐ none displayed

Additional Notes:

☐ **Easily distracted**
- ☐ external distractions
  - ☐ auditory:
    - ☐ talking
    - ☐ music
    - ☐ noises
      - ☐ ongoing
      - ☐ intermittent
  - ☐ visual
    - ☐ movement in room
    - ☐ stationary objects
    - ☐ view out window
- ☐ internal distractions
  - ☐ appears preoccupied with internal thoughts
  - ☐ verbosity and extraneous comments
  - ☐ physical discomfort (e.g., headaches, pain)

Additional Notes:

APPENDIX 2-E
Client Response to Assessment

Name _____

Date: _____

As I am interested in knowing how you were feeling following the demands of today's testing, please take a few minutes to answer the following questions and mail within three days after your evaluation.

1. Please describe your physical and mental energy levels throughout the remainder of the testing day.

2. Please describe your level of productivity regarding completion of your typical daily demands following the testing.

3. Please describe your mood and desire to interact with family, friends, or colleagues following the assessment.

4. Please list any and all concerns you had following the completion of this evaluation process.

Clinician Note

It is helpful to obtain information from your client regarding how he or she felt, physically and mentally, following the demands of the testing situation. The above questions are intentionally vague to avoid suggesting possible responses to the client; however, the client's documentation of fatigue and energy levels, emotional response, and ability to accomplish daily living or work tasks may add valuable support to your evaluation results and interpretive comments. Lastly, by requesting the client to mail this response questionnaire within three days following the evaluation, you will informally assess prospective memory.

APPENDIX 2-F
Sample Evaluation Segments

ATTENTION AND INFORMATION-PROCESSING SPEED AND ACCURACY

Based on Eric's reported concerns, as well as his description of an extremely hectic work environment, information-processing skills in both the auditory and visual modalities were assessed both with and without distractions. As an objective measure of Eric's information processing rate and as an indirect assessment of his sustained attention, cognitive flexibility, and working memory, the *Paced Auditory Serial Addition Test* (PASAT) (Gronwall, 1977) was administered. This test requires the skills of rapid addition of single digits presented verbally and immediate recall of previously stated numbers. Eric scored 42 (mean = 46; s.d. = 6) with an averaged processing time of 3.4 seconds. Despite his adequate performance, the constancy and speed of the stimulation appeared to be extremely frustrating for Eric. He experienced difficulty with resuming concentration when he lost pace with the taped presentation. Eric reported irritation with the task and had the desire to turn off the tape recorder. It is possible that, when Eric experiences such sensory overload at his job, his low frustration tolerance may interfere with his performance.

To assess speed and accuracy of information-processing in the visual or reading modality, an informal measure involving scanning for multiple elements within a page of information was utilized. Eric performed with 98% accuracy with talk radio in the background, demonstrating good selective attention and attention to detail. A more integrated processing test that was administered, which required reading rather than just scanning, was the *Speed and Capacity of Language Processing Test* (SCOLP) (Baddeley, Emslie, & Smith, 1992). On this test, Eric was required to silently read a list of sentences and determine if they were meaningful as quickly as possible. Meaning determination relies on common sense rather than higher level reasoning. Eric performed with 98% accuracy, and scored in the 66th percentile for speed. Interestingly, when talk radio was introduced into the background, Eric's speed was drastically reduced, such that he scored in the 19th percentile. Clearly, his reduced ability to inhibit distractions interferes with performance on tasks and may account for reduced productivity and his reported feelings of not "keeping everything together." Future therapy will target speed of processing, frustration tolerance, and both sustained and selective attention as they impact Eric's ability to comprehend, integrate, and recall complex, lengthy and detailed information presented in both the auditory and visual modalities, as necessary for successful work performance.

VERBAL EXPRESSION

Evelyn demonstrated functional verbal skills with good speech intelligibility; however, difficulties with higher level word retrieval, thought formulation, and thought organization were periodically demonstrated during conversational speech, interrupting fluent verbal thought expression. Specifically, while discussing her opinion on several controversial issues, pauses in her speech indicated thought delays and word-retrieval difficulties. Furthermore, she periodically became tangential in her discussion and lost her train of thought. Still, she displayed good thought elaboration and explanation of her ideas. While stuttering was not observed during relaxed conversational speech, under testing pressure during the timed Naming Subtest of the *Test of Adolescent/Adult Word Finding* (TAWF) (German, 1990), Evelyn stuttered on 32% of the words. Both speech blocks and part-word repetitions were observed. On the *TAWF* (German, 1990), which is an objective measure of word-retrieval skills, Evelyn objectively scored in the normal range for speed and accuracy of naming when compared to others in the 60–80 age range. Such performance should be interpreted with caution, however, since if Evelyn would be compared to others in the age range of 40–59 (in which she would have been just 3 months ago), she would have been categorized as a slow, although accurate, namer. Again, higher level word-retrieval delays were observed in natural conversation, compromising her ability to rapidly retrieve specific words. Additionally, extraneous verbalizations indicating word-retrieval difficulty were noted on 7% of target words. Reduced word access was documented on the *Scales of Cognitive Ability for Traumatic Brain Injury* (SCATBI) (Adamovich & Henderson, 1992) such that Evelyn provided 9 to 11 words beginning with a specific letter when allowed to brainstorm for 1 minute (14 and above is considered within normal range). Future therapy will address these speech and language areas to enhance Evelyn's ability to communicate effectively and fluently.

AUDITORY PROCESSING AND COMPREHENSION

Auditory processing skills were assessed informally on tests involving directions of increasing length and complexity. On the Oral Directions Subtest of the *Detroit Test of Learning Aptitude—2* (Hammill, 1985), which requires retention of lengthy, detailed directions, Caroline demonstrated the ability to follow two-step directions comprised of three to four details. Difficulty was displayed when the number of details or directions increased. Specifically, when provided three-step directions, Caroline accurately executed all parts of the direction with 72% accuracy. Four-step directions were too difficult to retain in order to follow. For paragraph length information, Caroline was verbally presented with information on the Recall Subtest of the *Scales of Cognitive Ability for Traumatic Brain Injury* (SCATBI) (Adamovich & Henderson, 1992). Caroline demonstrated good processing of information of brief paragraph length. Fluctuating cerebral efficiency, which is characteristic of people with traumatic brain injuries, may account for Caroline's reported periodic difficulty with taking in information while listening, and needing to "repeat it back to myself to make sense of it." Future therapy will target underlying attention and memory impairments as they impact Caroline's ability to comprehend, integrate, and recall complex, lengthier information necessary for new learning. This impacts her success with social interactions and independent completion of daily and work-related tasks.

READING PROCESSING AND COMPREHENSION

As discussed previously, Ken demonstrated accurate comprehension of sentence-length information on the *Speed and Capacity of Language Processing Test* (SCOLP) (Baddeley, Emslie, & Smith 1992). Additionally, on a nonstandardized task of following written directions, Ken completed two-step directions with 94% accuracy. To assess reading decoding and comprehension skills at the paragraph level, the *Gray Oral Reading Test—Revised* (GORT-R) (Wiederholt & Bryant, 1986) was administered. Ken demonstrated adequate oral decoding skills for accuracy and rate, and self-corrected many errors. Response to multiple choice factual and inferential questions revealed difficulty with retention of facts and integration of information in order to make inferences. With paragraphs of 8 to 13 lines, Ken responded to questions with 60–80% accuracy. Performance improved to 100% for factual questions and 80% for inferential questions when Ken was permitted to refer back to the information to scan for answers. Therapy will target Ken's ability to comprehend, integrate, and retain functional information of personal relevance and appropriate complexity, necessary for new learning and increased independence with tasks completed preinjury.

MEMORY

Emma openly expressed her current concerns regarding her memory impairments and the resulting impact on her daily functioning. She reported both frustration and embarrassment when she forgets work-related details or prior events, stating, "This has eroded my confidence." Based on these reported difficulties, a variety of memory tests were administered to determine Emma's memory skills for different types of information. The *California Verbal Learning Test* (CVLT) (Delis, Kramer, Kaplan & Ober, 1987) was utilized to evaluate Emma's ability to recall, retain, and recognize a list of words following a time delay, as well as a distraction word list. Emma recalled a list of 16 words in four semantic categories, presented across five trials, with 84% accuracy. She independently and successfully utilized "semantic clustering" (i.e., consecutive recall of words from the same category) as a compensatory strategy to enhance recall of the word lists. In addition, she benefitted from repetition as she increased the total number of words recalled after each trial, indicating good learning potential. Furthermore, Emma recalled 15 of 16 words (94% accuracy) after a 20-minute delay, indicating a good ability to retain verbal information of word length over time.

Secondly, to evaluate Emma's prospective memory, which is defined as the ability to "remember to remember" (e.g., an appointment), the *Prospective Memory Screening* (PROMS) (Sohlberg & Mateer, 1989) was administered. Throughout the test, Emma was required to execute specific activities when provided an associative cue (e.g., "When I hold up this picture, you may leave the room") or a time cue (e.g., "Write your name on this page in two minutes"). In addition, Emma completed a memory questionnaire and basic math problems on paper as distractors. Overall, Emma successfully utilized the associative cues to complete two of three required tasks and the time cues to complete three of four required tasks. Her score of 5 indicates a borderline impairment in her ability to perform specific tasks at designated times. This suggests Emma may have mild-to-moderate difficulties remembering to initiate and complete daily living tasks in the naturally distracting environment, such as paying bills, returning a phone call, or taking medication. In fact, similar difficulties were reported by her. To summarize, Emma displayed excellent verbal memory skills and use of compensatory strategies for word recall tasks, yet demonstrated memory difficulties for lengthier, functional information. Therefore, therapy will target underlying attention, as it impacts memory encoding and storage of functional verbal information of increased length and complexity. In addition, therapy will address prospective memory skills and further develop useful compensatory strategies to enhance Emma's memory function as it impacts her daily living and work performance.

WRITING

Ellen reported significant difficulty with functional writing skills both for school and daily tasks. During an informal assessment, she was required to discuss the pros, cons, and her opinion regarding a controversial issue of her choice. While expressing some anxiety with the task, Ellen was able to attempt it. Significantly delayed thought formulation and expression were demonstrated; however, her initial outlining of pros and cons assisted with stimulating thought formulation. Difficulty with paragraph formulation, cohesion, sentence transition, word choice, and spelling were documented. Ellen demonstrated consistent self-monitoring skills needed to correct perseverative letter errors which resulted in misspelled words. Writing skills will require further improvement for academic and long-term vocational goals. In addition, although no limitations in motoric ability were displayed, Ellen's writing skills are not considered functional from a cognitive perspective for such multiprocessing daily tasks as taking notes, taking telephone directions, and writing a telephone message.

MATH

Functional math skills were assessed utilizing subtests of the *Scholastic Abilities Test for Adults* (SATA) (Bryant, Patton, & Dunn, 1991). Problems on the Math Calculation subtest addressed the areas of addition, subtraction, multiplication, division, fractions, decimals, and others related to geometry and algebra. Joe completed 94% of the problems accurately, scoring in the 84th percentile. Due to reduced speed of processing, however, he did not complete all of the problems in the time allotted. When required to apply computation skills to solve word problems on the Math Application subtest, Joe demonstrated good integration of skills and strategies to determine answers with 92% accuracy, scoring in the 91st percentile. Still, he required twice the amount of allotted time to complete the problems. Lastly, when completing functional math problems on an informal worksheet, he scored 90%. Overall, Joe displayed accurate performance on the math portions of the assessment; however, reduced speed of processing interfered with his ability to efficiently compute the answers. Additionally, he reported significant frustration with his inability to compute higher level math problems as he did preinjury, as a math professor.

EXECUTIVE FUNCTIONING

To gain understanding of Ralph's work environment and responsibilities, obtain a functional assessment of his work demands and concerns, and supplement objective test measures, a work visit was made by this therapist. The *Profile of Executive Control System* (PRO-EX) (Braswell, Hartry, Hoornbeek, Johansen, Johnson, Schultz, & Sohlberg, 1992) was utilized to rate executive functioning skills using the work environment as the observation site. Ralph demonstrated mild-to- moderate difficulty with goal selection, planning, task execution and completion, and time sense (awareness and organization). Organization of information and tasks was more moderately to severely impaired and further complicated by attention and memory limitations. For example, Ralph received a return call from a therapist to whom he had made a referral. At that time he was unable to locate the sheet of information needed to discuss the client. He indicated he would call her back when he located the sheet; however, he did not write a note to himself to return the call. He appeared quite frustrated with not being able to locate the information stating, "I just had it." It became apparent that reductions in organization, memory, attention to detail, and self-monitoring skills are severely impacting Ralph's ability to efficiently and successfully manage his business. Ralph was extremely willing to follow suggested strategies, which were provided for immediate relief, as well as to assess Ralph's openness to modifying his environment and changing his preinjury methods. Based on his initial responsiveness, it is believed that Ralph would benefit significantly from instruction on strategy use (in addition to skill relearning) to compensate for his difficulties.

SUMMARY AND RECOMMENDATIONS

In summary, Margaret demonstrated strengths in the areas of pragmatics, verbal expression, basic auditory processing and comprehension, word retrieval, reasoning and problem solving, complex reading comprehension and retention, and basic math. She displayed limitations in the areas of: prospective memory; retention, recall, and speed of processing information in the visual modality; sustained, selective, alternating, and divided attention skills; and frustration tolerance for challenging tasks that require the use of several language and cognitive skills simultaneously. Based on the evaluation results and Margaret's corresponding self-reports and concerns, it is recommended that she receive individual cognitive-language therapy 2 to 4 hours per week with an emphasis on the following goals:

1. Improve complex attention skills including sustained, alternating, selective, and divided attention, as these impact active therapy participation, tolerance for distractions, and consistent higher level communication functioning at home and work.

2. Maximize functional memory skills by targeting prospective memory and underlying attention and information organization, as well as by developing additional effective compensatory memory strategies that would be useful to Margaret at home and work.

3. Improve auditory and visual processing speed and accuracy for adequate comprehension of functional information of increasing length and complexity, through structured practice and development of effective compensatory strategies.

APPENDIX 2-G
Vocational Recommendations

COGNITIVE STRENGTHS AND LIMITATIONS, AS THEY RELATE TO POTENTIAL JOB PLACEMENT

SUMMARY OF STRENGTHS:

Overall, Madison demonstrates excellent skills in the following areas: verbal expression, pragmatic skills, written expression, math computation and application, as well as creativity and a strong motivation to do her best. Therefore, a job working with others is recommended given Madison's strong social and interpersonal skills. Additionally, a job involving interaction with others would provide emotional stimulation and provide necessary feedback for task completion.

LIMITATIONS IN DETAIL:

Information Processing:

Listening: Madison displays functional, basic auditory processing skills; however, underlying memory impairments and concentration difficulties interfere with her ability to quickly process and comprehend increasing amounts of information, such as complex, lengthy verbal directions. *She would benefit from written job instructions in a simple step-by-step form.*

Reading: Madison has the ability to read basic paragraph-length information, yet at a reduced speed of processing. *Brief instructions with written reminders are recommended. Jobs involving lengthy reading such as working in a library or scripted telemarketing are not recommended.*

Complex Attention: Madison demonstrates a reduced ability to concentrate and maintain her attention amidst distractions, which interferes with task completion. *Therefore, a large, noisy work environment is not recommended. Initially, a fairly quiet setting with minimal distractions would be best, such as bookkeeping for a small store or working in a small tree nursery or flower shop.*

Memory and Learning: As complex attention skills underlie memory and learning, Madison displays additional limitations in the area of encoding, storing, and recalling learned information. Repetition, structure, and use of compensatory strategies learned in individual therapy will be strongly needed for successful job completion. For example, *Madison should write down specific information, such as her work schedule, to enhance accurate recall.*

Distractibility: Madison demonstrates significant difficulty with any type of environmental distraction such as a radio playing, people talking, telephone ringing, and so on. Typically, Madison successfully completes basic verbal directions independently until distractions are present. This is the area that causes the most difficulty for Madison. *In a job situation, directions would need to be shortened and tasks would need to be clearly defined.* The work environment and the amount of distractions in the potential work environment should be considered to promote future job success. *A sheltered work setting is not being recommended, yet if possible, environmental noises should be kept to a minimum.*

Stress and Frustration Tolerance: Madison appears to be dedicated and determined to perform at her very best with all therapy tasks. She is a very focused person; however, she becomes easily discouraged if tasks are too difficult. Madison attempts to focus herself and she tends to complete tasks the way she did prior to her accident. However, without successful use of strategies, some level of failure is usually evident. *To achieve success, Madison must have assistance with the development and implementation of compensatory strategies (refer to self-monitoring section of this report for further information). Also, it may be beneficial to seek further information from her psychologist regarding strategies for stress reduction.*

Functional Problem Solving: Madison's complex problem-solving skills are inconsistent. Although she demonstrates good reasoning skills on most structured treatment tasks, functionally Madison often does not independently think through a problematic situation prior to reacting. *In a job setting, it would be beneficial to closely monitor this skill area and provide positive, corrective feedback if necessary. Also, providing Madison with ample time to solve her work-related problems will be of utmost importance for her success.*

Time Management: This is an area in which Madison will require strict supervision and assistance in the development and implementation of compensatory strategies. As several home strategies were implemented for time management skills, a review of these would be recommended before vocational strategies are developed. *Work-related strategies should be somewhat similar to the implemented home strategies for a positive response to occur.*

Self-Monitoring: Self-monitoring skills are the ability to correct one's mistakes from information learned within the environment. As stated previously, Madison ineffectively relies on her preinjury abilities and lifestyle to handle daily situations. It is believed that this will occur in the work setting and feedback will be necessary. Madison requires assistance to learn and utilize new learning systems. Her opinions and ideas were very resourceful in the development of her home compensatory strategies. *For future vocational success, strategies* must *be designed to meet her specific needs.*

In conclusion, it is our professional opinion that Madison would initially benefit from a structured part-time job (a maximum of 15-20 hours per week). The specific job would need to accommodate her current level of capabilities and rehabilitation needs. As therapy addresses her deficit areas, her overall potential to work will increase and improvements in job readiness skills will be determined. If you have any further questions, please do not hesitate to call our office.

APPENDIX 2-H
Standardized Tests for Use with Clients with Mild-to-Moderate TBI

The Adolescent Word Test (Zachman, Barrett, Huisingh, Orman, & Blagden, 1989)
Linguisystems
1-800-PRO-IDEA
3100 4th Avenue, E. Moline, IL 61214

Associate Learning Subtest of the *Wechsler Memory Scale—3* (Wechsler, 1997)
The Psychological Corporation
1-800-211-8378
555 Academic Court, San Antonio, TX 78204-2498

Boston Naming Test (Kaplan, Goodglass, & Weintraub, 1983)
Lea & Febiger
600 S. Washington Square, Philadelphia, PA 19106

California Verbal Learning Test (CVLT) (Delis, Kramer, Kaplan, & Ober 1987)
The Psychological Corporation
1-800-211-8378
555 Academic Court, San Antonio, TX 78204-2498

Clinical Evaluation of Language Functions—3 (CELF-3) (Semel, Wiig & Secord, 1996)
The Psychological Corporation
1-800-211-8378
555 Academic Court, San Antonio, TX 78204-2498

Detroit Tests of Learning Aptitude—2 (DTLA–2) (Hammill, 1985)
PRO-ED
1-800-897-3202
8700 Shoal Creek Boulevard, Austin, TX 78757-6897

Discourse Comprehension Test (Brookshire & Nicholas, 1993)
The Psychological Corporation
1-800-211-8378
555 Academic Court, San Antonio, TX 78204-2498

Gray Oral Reading Tests—Revised (Gort–R) (Wiederholt & Bryant, 1986)
PRO-ED
1-800-897-3202
8700 Shoal Creek Boulevard, Austin, TX 78757-6897

Kaufman Test of Educational Achievement (KTEA) (Kaufman & Kaufman, 1985)
American Guidance Service, Inc.
1-800-328-2560
P.O. Box 99, Circle Pines, MN 55014-1796

Learning Efficiency Test II (LET–II) (Webster, 1992)
Academic Therapy Publishing
1-800-422-7249
20 Commercial Boulevard, Novato, CA 94949

Paced Auditory Serial Addition Test (PASAT) (Gronwall, 1977)
  Association for Neurological Research and Development
  1420 S. Meridian, Suite A, Puyallup, WA 98371

Profile of Executive Control System (PRO-EX) (Braswell, Hartry, Hoornbeek, Johansen, Johnson, Schultz, & Sohlberg, 1992)
  Association for Neurological Research and Development
  1420 S. Meridian, Suite A, Puyallup, WA 98371

Prospective Memory Screening (PROMS) (Sohlberg & Mateer, 1989)
  Association for Neurological Research and Development
  1420 S. Meridian, Suite A, Puyallup, WA 98371

Rivermead Behavioral Memory Test (Wilson, Cockburn, & Baddeley, 1985)
  Thames Valley
  7-9 The Green, Flempton
  Bury St. Edmunds, Suffolk, 1P286EL ENGLAND

Ross Information Processing Assessment—Second Edition (Ross-Swain, 1996)
  PRO-ED
  1-800-897-3202
  8700 Shoal Creek Boulevard, Austin, TX 78757-6897

Scales of Cognitive Ability for Traumatic Brain Injury (SCATBI) (Adamovich & Henderson, 1992)
  The Riverside Publishing Company
  1-800-323-9540
  8420 Bryn Mawr Avenue, Chicago, IL 60631

Scholastic Abilities Test for Adults (SATA) (Bryant, Patton, & Dunn, 1991)
  PRO-ED
  1-800-897-3202
  8700 Shoal Creek Boulevard, Austin, TX 78757-6897

The Speed and Capacity of Language Processing Test (SCOLP) (Baddeley, Emslie, & Smith 1992)
  Thames Valley
  7-9 The Green, Flempton
  Bury St. Edmunds, Suffolk, 1P286EL ENGLAND

Test of Adolescent/Adult Word Finding (TAWF) (German, 1990)
  PRO-ED
  1-800-897-3202
  8700 Shoal Creek Boulevard, Austin, TX 78757-6897

The Test of Everyday Attention (TEA) (Robertson, Ward, Ridgeway, & Nimmo-Smith, 1994)
  Thames Valley
  7-9 The Green, Flempton
  Bury St. Edmunds, Suffolk, 1P286EL ENGLAND

Woodcock-Johnson Test of Cognitive Ability (Woodcock & Johnson, 1989)
  The Riverside Publishing Company
  1-800-323-9540
  8420 Bryn Mawr Avenue, Chicago, IL 60631

SOURCES OF ADDITIONAL INFORMATION

Neuropsychological Evaluation

Acimovic, M., Keatley, M., & Lemmon, J. (1993). The importance of qualitative indicators in the assessment of mild brain injury. *The Journal of Cognitive Rehabilitation, 11*(6), 8–14.

Kay, T. (1993). Neuropsychological treatment of mild traumatic brain injury. *The Journal of Head Trauma Rehabilitation, 8*(3), 74–85.

Kay, T., Harrington, D. E., Adams, R., Anderson, T., Berrol, S., Cicerone, K., Dahlberg, C., Gerber, D., Goka, R., Harley, P., Hilt, J., Horn, L., Lehmkuhl, D., & Malec, J. (1993). Definition of mild traumatic brain injury. *The Journal of Head Trauma Rehabilitation, 8*(3), 86–87.

Lamport-Hughes, N. (1995). Learning potential and other predictors of cognitive rehabilitation. *The Journal of Cognitive Rehabilitation, 13*(4), 16–21.

Lewkowicz, S. S., & Whitton, J. L. (1995). A new inventory for exploring neuropsychological change resulting from brain injury. *The Journal of Cognitive Rehabilitation, 13*(1), 8–20.

Uomoto, J. M. (1991). Evaluation of neuropsychological status after traumatic brain injury. In D. Beukelman & K. Yorkston (Eds.), *Communication disorders following traumatic brain injury: Management of cognitive, language, and motor impairments* (pp. 75–101). Austin, TX: Pro-Ed.

Speech-Language Assessment

Depoy, E. (1992). A comparison of standardized and observational assessment. *The Journal of Cognitive Rehabilitation, 10*(1), 30–32.

Ellmo, W. (1995). Assessment issues in mild TBI. *Advance for Speech-Language Pathologists and Audiologists, 5*(34), 17.

Frank, E. M., & Barrineau, S. (1996). Current speech-language assessment protocols for adults with traumatic brain injury. *Journal of Medical Speech-Language Pathology, 4*(2), 81–101.

Iskowitz, M. (1996). Testing in TBI: Formal and informal mix needed to meet patient needs. *Advance for Speech-Language Pathologists and Audiologists, 6*(35), 6–7, 10.

CHAPTER 3

Treatment of Mild-to-Moderate Traumatic Brain Injury

FACILITATING A POSITIVE THERAPEUTIC RELATIONSHIP

To be successful in treating individuals who have sustained a mild or moderate TBI, clinicians must develop a positive therapeutic relationship and utilize a functional, personalized therapy approach. Although it is most therapeutic to utilize highly functional and personally relevant therapy tasks along with a supportive, empowering therapy approach with any communication-disordered population, it is essential with the mildly-to-moderately traumatic brain injured population for the following reasons. First, their awareness is usually more intact than in people who are more severely brain injured. These clients are aware of their skill limitations, the impact on their daily living, and how the clinician establishes rapport with them. A variety of psychological and self-esteem issues, which include depression regarding loss of functioning and reduced self-confidence, often result from having this awareness (Kay, 1993). As a consequence, clients often come to rely on their speech-language pathologist to assist them in regaining their cognitive-language skills, and, in turn, their self-esteem and ability to return to preinjury activities. This requires development of a therapeutic relationship that is both supportive and goal-oriented.

Second, emotional issues are often documented in this population, possibly stemming from their heightened awareness, as well as the fact that they are often treated as if they have no difficulties because they look "normal" physically and often display appropriate social skills. As a result of this, as well as the fact that deficits are often quite subtle, there is an expectation by others (including family, friends, coworkers, boss, and self) that they should be functioning as they did preinjury. This may create stress, frustration, and feelings of inadequacy, which are often reported by both the clients and their psychologists or social workers. By being sensitive to these issues through a positive therapeutic relationship, progress with cognitive-language skills can continue to be made in therapy. Finally, adults with mild-to-moderate TBI have increased potential to return to independent living and a work or school environment. To maximize generalization and successful reintegration, therapy must be as functional and similar to the challenges of these natural environments as possible.

To facilitate a positive, productive therapeutic relationship with this client population, a variety of techniques can be utilized (see Appendix 3-A). These techniques should be incorporated into therapy sessions not only in the initial session, but throughout the duration of treatment. They are not presented in any hierarchical fashion as they are all equally important at various times during the therapeutic relationship. When the clients feel they can trust you with their questions and concerns, you are interested in them as people, you value their input, and therapy is being directed by their concerns and goals (with your guidance), clients are more likely to be invested in their therapy, listen to you, be motivated by you, and be empowered by you, which will increase their chances of success.

INTEREST SURVEY

To promote increased understanding of the client as a unique individual and thereby further develop the therapeutic relationship, an interest survey can be utilized (see Appendix 3-B). This provides the clinician with a global understanding of the client and what is meaningful to him or her. Keep in mind that you are not treating an isolated cognitive skill, but rather an entire person who is experiencing difficulty resuming his or her life as a result of cognitive-language limitations. The survey in Appendix 3-B also can be utilized when creating therapy tasks, making them more personally relevant and motivating to a particular client. Specifically, it provides ideas for therapy tasks and interactions that are sensitive to and respectful of the client's unique perspective. It is best to have the client complete the survey at home and then bring it back to discuss with you during the next treatment session. In addition to providing you with familiarity with the person, it tells the client that what he or she thinks and feels is important to the treating clinician, thus furthering a positive therapeutic relationship.

IMPORTANCE OF RELEVANT THERAPY TASKS

In addition to developing a therapeutic relationship, our second criterion for a successful therapy outcome is to provide functional, personally relevant therapy tasks. When planning treatment, tasks must be presented at an adult level and comprised of age-appropriate content so as not to insult the client by being either too simplistic or too difficult. For tasks to be functional and personally relevant, they must be as related to the client's life and future goals as possible. Some ways to achieve this include explaining the rationale of each therapy task as it relates to the client's limitations and skill enhancement, incorporating information generated from the Personal Interest Survey in Appendix 3-B (e.g., using reading material on a topic of interest to the client), and requesting feedback from the client by asking "How do you think you did?" By eliciting the client's opinion, you increase his or her feelings of involvement in the therapy process, as well as gain information regarding the client's level of awareness and expectations of him- or herself. To obtain specific information, try to elicit feedback regarding level of task difficulty and its applicability to the client's personal life and outcome goals.

In addition to being personally relevant and meaningful, therapy should also be highly functional to the client's current and future goal activities. Such an approach will facilitate increased generalization to a personally relevant setting, enhance the meaningfulness of therapy to the client, and result in a faster, lasting progression in therapy. When task planning, consider the current demands which the client reports as difficult, whether they are in the home, work, or school environments. When possible, tasks should then simulate these environments. For example, material from a school text can be utilized to practice reading comprehension skills, vocabulary skills, and use of compensatory strategies. In addition, listening skills could be targeted using an outline of text material during an instructional therapy session. In the same way, simulating a noisy work environment during attention tasks using talk radio would be functional for a client who is currently in, or hopes to return to, that type of job environment. Making an initial home, work, or school visit can be highly instructive in helping the clinician understand its cognitive demands on the client and his or her resulting difficulties. From this perspective, functional tasks and useful, individualized compensatory strategies can be developed. If a desired outcome setting has not been identified, it is advisable to target foundational cognitive-language skills to enhance a client's potential to return to work or school.

RATIONALE FOR SELECTED SKILLS TO TARGET

The therapy tasks in Chapters 4–8 can be utilized in two ways. First, they may be used to address foundational cognitive-language skills before a discharge environment has been determined. Second, they may be modified to promote specific work- or school-related skills the client needs for either on-the-job or academic success. Although each TBI is unique and each client requires individually tailored treatment, several cognitive-language skill areas are typically impaired to varying degrees in the mild-to-moderate TBI population. These limitations are often found to significantly interfere with daily living, vocational, and academic demands. Thus, we chose the five cognitive-language areas of:

■ Complex attention

■ Functional and prospective memory

■ Higher level communication skills

■ Auditory and visual information processing

■ Executive functioning

For each skill section, the skill will be defined and the impact of related cognitive-language impairments will be explained. A list of functional implications of the impaired skill on performance in the home, work, and school environments follows. Next, specific tasks to address the skill area will be presented along with the following:

1. Suggestions on how to increase the complexity level through hierarchical procedures;

2. A list of other cognitive-language skills that may be addressed simultaneously, by utilizing suggested task modifications; and

3. A list of specific, optional performance measures to assist clinicians in thorough, objective documentation.

To promote generalization and skill maintenance, home tasks and ideas for further stimulation will be provided. Finally, suggestions for families and caregivers will be offered to facilitate understanding of their family members with TBI and to further promote your clients' success through their families' support, sensitivity, and insight.

ADDITIONAL THERAPY RESOURCES

We have found the following sources of information useful in planning personally relevant and interesting therapy for our clients. Each resource can be utilized with the task formats presented in the subsequent therapy task chapters.

Books

Goodwin, P. (1992). *How everyday things work*. Portland, OR: J. Weston Walch.

Scott, M. (1993). *Of many times and cultures*. Portland, OR: J. Weston Walch.

Seidenberg, P. L. (1991). *Reading, writing, and studying strategies: An integrated curriculum*. Gaithersburg, MD: Aspen Publishers.

Whimby, A., & Lochhead, J. (1986). *Problem solving and comprehension*. Hillsdale, NJ: Lawrence Erlbaum Associates.

Sample Magazines of Personal Interest to Clients

Reader's Digest
Prevention
Consumer Reports
U.S. News and World Report
Sports Illustrated
Smart Money
Parents
Self
Good Housekeeping

Sample Televised Programs to Videotape

Prime Time Live (ABC)
Dateline (NBC)
60 Minutes (CBS)
Turning Point (ABC)
20-20 (ABC)
Nightline (ABC)
World News (NBC, CBS, ABC, CNN)

Sample Radio Programs to Audiotape

National Public Radio
Talk shows
News

APPENDIX 3-A

Techniques for Developing a Therapeutic Relationship with the Client

1. Discuss topics of personal interest, hobbies, etc.; encourage the client to talk about him- or herself.

2. Respond to questions of concern with genuine care and without patronizing the client.

3. Solicit client's viewpoints, insights, and opinions; inform him or her that you have learned something new.

4. Ask follow-up questions over time regarding personal events of importance to the client.

5. Discuss general topics and request the client's perspective (facilitates orientation and validates his or her thoughts and feelings).

6. Make therapy a collaborative effort by involving the client in goal setting, task selection, and home tasks.

7. Respond to frustration with sensitive, supportive comments and objective information to convey a realistic, yet optimistic viewpoint.

8. Smile often.

9. Be a good listener.

10. Take advantage of opportunities to point out the client's positive qualities, actions, and comments to enhance his or her self-confidence which is typically compromised after an injury. Help the client to feel good about him- or herself!

11. Provide intermittent positive feedback on task performance in an adult-like manner (e.g., "That seemed easy for you." "You did well on that." "You improved by 20%." "You required less cueing from me").

Note: These techniques are not presented in any specific order and may be presented to the client in any order at any time in the therapeutic process.

APPENDIX 3-B
Personal Interest Survey

1. List several of your hobbies.

   1.

   2.

   3.

2. Are you currently involved in these activities? Why or why not?

3. List the types of magazines, movies, books, television programs, and music you enjoy.

4. List several topics of discussion that are of interest to you.

5. Name and discuss two people who have had a significant impact on your life. In what ways have they influenced you?

6. In what ways are you hoping therapy will assist you?

SOURCES OF ADDITIONAL INFORMATION

Treatment

Adamovich, B. (1991). Cognition, language, attention, and information processing following closed head injury. In J. S. Kreutzer & P. H. Wehman (Eds.), *Cognitive rehabilitation for persons with traumatic brain injury: A functional approach* (pp. 75–86). Baltimore, MD: Paul H. Brookes.

Haarbauer-Krupa, J., Henry, K., Szekeres, S., & Ylvisaker, M. (1985). Cognitive rehabilitation therapy: Late stages of recovery. In M. Ylvisaker (Ed.), *Head injury rehabilitation: Children and adolescents* (pp. 311–340). San Diego, CA: College-Hill Press.

Honsinger, M., & Yorkston, K. (1991). Compensation for memory and related disorders following traumatic brain injury. In D. Beukelman & K. Yorkston (Eds.), *Communication disorders following traumatic brain injury: Management of cognitive, language, and motor impairments* (pp. 103–121). Austin, TX: Pro-Ed.

Kennedy, M., & DeRuyter, F. (1991). Cognitive and language bases for communication disorders. In D. Beukelman & K. Yorkston (Eds.), *Communication disorders following traumatic brain injury: Management of cognitive, language, and motor impairments* (pp. 123–190). Austin, TX: Pro-Ed.

Nelson, N., & Schwentor, B. (1991). Reading and writing disorders. In D. Beukelman & K. Yorkston (Eds.), *Communication disorders following traumatic brain injury: Management of cognitive, language, and motor impairments* (pp. 191–249). Austin, TX: Pro-Ed.

Parente, R., & DiCesare, A. (1991). Retraining memory: Theory, evaluation, and applications. In J. S. Kreutzer & P. H. Wehman (Eds.), *Cognitive rehabilitation for persons with traumatic brain injury: A functional approach* (pp. 147–162). Baltimore, MD: Paul H. Brookes.

Pepin, M, Loranger, M., & Benoit, G. (1995). Efficiency of cognitive training: Review and prospects. *The Journal of Cognitive Rehabilitation*, 13(4), 8–14.

Wilson, B. (1987). *Rehabilitation of memory*. New York: The Guilford Press.

CHAPTER 4

Treating Complex Attention Impairments

DEFINITION

Attention

A fundamental skill required for new learning and successful cognitive functioning that allows one to focus on incoming stimuli. In their treatment model, Mateer and Moore-Sohlberg (1992) describe five types of attention:

1. **Focused:** Able to respond discretely to specific visual, auditory, and tactile stimulation

2. **Sustained:** Able to maintain consistent behavioral response during continuous or repetitive activity

3. **Selective:** Able to select and maintain cognitive focus in the presence of internal or external distractions or other competing stimuli (distractibility)

4. **Alternating:** Capable of mental flexibility that allows for moving between tasks that have different cognitive requirements (shifting attention)

5. **Divided:** Able to simultaneously respond to multiple stimuli (completing two tasks at the same time)

Specific to the mild-to-moderate TBI population, impairments in this skill area may manifest themselves in difficulties such as:

Compromised ability to maintain focused attention due to fatigue, pain, or sensory overload

■ Reduced ability to inhibit distractions when completing tasks

■ Inability to shift focus from one task to another

■ Difficulty completing two tasks simultaneously

OTHER CONTRIBUTING COGNITIVE IMPAIRMENTS

Cognitive impairments that may be seen in people with mild-to-moderate TBI that may result in **attentional** difficulties:

Difficulties with:	May lead to:
1. Insight	Difficulty with awareness of the need to use compensatory attention strategies
2. Self-monitoring	Difficulty consistently utilizing compensatory attention strategies

FUNCTIONAL IMPLICATIONS OF ATTENTIONAL IMPAIRMENTS

The following is a list of many of the abilities needed for successful functioning in the natural environments of home, work, and school. Impairments in complex attention skills in people with mild-to-moderate TBI may compromise performance in these functional environments. You are encouraged to explore these and other related activities with your clients to create functional and personally relevant therapy tasks and to maximize carryover of therapeutic gains to the natural environment.

Since attention underlies all cognitive-language skill areas and the majority of functional tasks, only a few primary examples have been provided to assist you in understanding the functional impact of attention deficits and to stimulate creative thinking to generate similar implications that are more personally relevant for your specific client.

In the Home

Ability to...

- **Sustain attention to complete lengthy home tasks**

  Examples:

  Organize home budget

  Reconcile checking account

  Organize personal papers and documents

  Pay monthly bills

- **Selectively inhibit attention to internal and external distractions in order to successfully complete home tasks**

  Examples:

  Complete business telephone calls with children playing in background or adults talking in background

  Work on personal computer program with television or radio on in background

- **Alternate attention between two different home tasks**

  Examples:

  Alternate between cooking dinner and responding to children's questions regarding homework

  Alternate between doing laundry and making cookies

- **Divide attention in order to focus on two or more home tasks simultaneously**

  Examples:

Reorganize closet while planning your day in your mind

Sort mail while talking on the telephone socially

At Work

Ability to...

■ **Sustain attention to complete lengthy job tasks**

Examples:

Prepare a written proposal

Concentrate during a meeting

Remain attentive throughout the work day

Type a lengthy document on the computer

■ **Selectively inhibit attention to internal and external distractions in order to successfully complete work tasks.**

Examples:

Review memos and work-related mail amid telephones ringing and people talking

Focus on current work task without thinking about your afternoon presentation

■ **Alternate attention between two different job tasks**

Examples:

Type document on computer and respond to incoming phone calls

Record inventory and respond to employee questions and concerns

■ **Divide attention in order to focus on two or more work tasks simultaneously**

Examples:

Simultaneously review typed document for both content and typographical errors

Audit balance sheet for accurate number entry, as well as balance of account

At School

Ability to...

■ **Sustain attention to complete lengthy school tasks**

Examples:

Pay close attention during a class or lecture

Read a text chapter

Complete a writing assignment

Remain attentive throughout the school day

Stay focused during an exam

■ **Selectively inhibit attention to internal and external distractions in order to successfully complete school tasks.**

Examples:

Work on assignment in library amid others' whispering

Concentrate during lecture despite background noises and talking

■ **Alternate attention between two different school tasks**

Examples:

Follow both sides of a debate

Read a text chapter and take notes or outline

■ **Divide attention in order to focus on two or more school tasks simultaneously**

Examples:

Listen to group members' comments while simultaneously writing responses

Take notes while listening to a lecture

In addition to the attention tasks provided in the following pages, you may utilize the information listed above to create unique therapy tasks that will be most meaningful for your client, depending on his or her goal environment. Please refer to the cover sheet for each task to assist you in addressing related skills simultaneously.

COMPENSATORY STRATEGIES

Select from the following list the attention strategies that would be most assistive to your clients and effectively utilized by them, considering their skill limitations and potential home, work, and school environments. It is recommended that these strategies be taught to the client and incorporated into the therapy sessions until the client is able to utilize them successfully and independently. Additionally, allow for practice of the specific strategy in the target environment to ensure successful carryover.

■ Know your attention limit and watch for indications that you need to take a break.

■ Set your watch or a timer to remind yourself to rest.

■ Determine what times during the day you are most attentive and maximize your efforts by completing demanding tasks at these times.

■ Be sure to get enough sleep on a consistent basis as fatigue will further reduce attentional capacities.

■ Keep a small notecard in view to cue you to stay focused (e.g., "Are you focused?" "What are you focusing on?" "What should you be focusing on?").

■ Use headphones or earplugs when in a noisy environment to reduce distractions.

■ Arrange your work environment to minimize visual distractions.

■ Write down distracting internal thoughts to address them at a later, more appropriate time.

■ Allow yourself time to adjust when changing tasks.

■ When changing tasks, verbalize what you are currently doing.

■ If you must do two things at once in order to be efficient, do one cognitive task and one automatic physical task that requires minimal cognitive effort.

■ Silently tell yourself "pay attention" while listening or reading.

COMPLEX ATTENTION TASKS

The first group of therapy tasks presented in Chapter 4 of this manual focuses primarily on the complex attention skills of sustained, selective, alternating, and divided attention. Additionally, as attention underlies all cognitive functioning, it is often impaired at some level in the mild-to-moderate TBI population. Therefore, ideas have been provided in Chapters 5 through 7 for addressing the various types of attention when utilizing modifications of the tasks created specifically for Information Processing, Functional Memory, and Word Retrieval/Thought Formulation. Refer to the section entitled "To Address the Related Skill of . . ." contained in the task cover sheet provided for every task in Chapters 5 through 7, to address attention more specifically, while simultaneously targeting other skill areas.

SUSTAINED ATTENTION TASK
UNSCRAMBLING WORDS

PURPOSE:

The purpose of this task is to improve the client's sustained attention for overall enhanced cognitive functioning.

DIRECTIONS:

Verbally present the client with scrambled words comprised of three to five letters. Request that the client retain the letters in short-term working memory and unscramble the letters in his or her mind to determine the target word.

TO INCREASE TASK DIFFICULTY:

1. Increase the number of letters provided.

2. Increase the rate of stimulus presentation.

3. Provide letters that spell more than one word and require the client to determine all words.

PRIMARY SKILLS TARGETED:

1. Sustained Attention

2. Alternating Attention

3. Working Memory Capacity and Efficiency

TO ADDRESS THE RELATED SKILL OF:	INCORPORATE THIS TASK MODIFICATION:
1. Speed of Processing	Impose time constraint (e.g., encourage client to determine words as quickly as possible)
2. Selective Attention	Complete task in a distracting environment (e.g., talk radio, others talking in background)

PERFORMANCE MEASURES:

Evaluate the following:

■ Ability to retain letters in short-term memory long enough to unscramble them

■ Ability to unscramble letters in mind

■ Percentage of words unscrambled correctly

■ Maximum number of letters able to retain and unscramble accurately

■ Length of time able to sustain attention to task before becoming fatigued

■ Effect of task modification(s) on performance (e.g., speed, distractions)

WORD LIST

3 LETTERS

1.	OZO	ZOO	37.	NTA	ANT, TAN	
2.	WOR	ROW	38.	IEP	PIE	
3.	EPA	PEA	39.	GDO	DOG, GOD	
4.	IBT	BIT	40.	BTA	BAT, TAB	
5.	FNI	FIN	41.	TPI	PIT, TIP	
6.	NED	DEN, END	42.	YBO	BOY	
7.	XFI	FIX	43.	EAC	ACE	
8.	RBI	RIB	44.	OTP	TOP, POT, OPT	
9.	PAG	GAP	45.	DSO	SOD	
10.	EIC	ICE	46.	SEU	SUE, USE	
11.	NTO	TON, NOT	47.	OHW	HOW, WHO	
12.	BTU	BUT, TUB	48.	GRU	RUG	
13.	APL	LAP, PAL	49.	RAF	FAR	
14.	TIW	WIT	50.	NMA	MAN	
15.	TVA	VAT	51.	NME	MEN	
16.	ORT	ROT	52.	NUS	SUN	
17.	EBE	BEE	53.	KYS	SKY	
18.	RIA	AIR	54.	YCO	COY	
19.	NVA	VAN	55.	SNO	SON	
20.	YJO	JOY	56.	NWI	WIN	
21.	NOE	ONE, EON	57.	YED	DYE	
22.	WNO	WON, NOW	58.	DER	RED	
23.	PNE	PEN	59.	TCA	CAT	
24.	HTU	HUT	60.	AYM	YAM, MAY	
25.	PSI	SIP	61.	OOB	BOO	
26.	IBD	BID	62.	PTA	PAT, TAP, APT	
27.	PTU	PUT	63.	ARJ	JAR	
28.	OCT	COT	64.	TAE	EAT, TEA, ATE	
29.	UTG	TUG, GUT	65.	SWA	SAW, WAS	
30.	GIF	FIG	66.	NBA	BAN, NAB	
31.	BJO	JOB	67.	AMD	DAM, MAD	
32.	YRC	CRY	68.	BAC	CAB	
33.	BWO	BOW	69.	UMG	MUG, GUM	
34.	WOT	TWO	70.	RTA	ART, RAT, TAR	
35.	ETI	TIE	71.	XAF	FAX	
36.	YEE	EYE	72.	AEL	ALE	

WORD LIST

3 LETTERS

73. ALY	LAY		**77.** LUF	FLU	
74. NPA	NAP, PAN		**78.** TFA	FAT	
75. NFU	FUN		**79.** LEM	ELM	
76. RFO	FOR		**80.** RYP	PRY	

WORD LIST

4 LETTERS

1. RTHU	HURT		21. LAED	DEAL, LEAD
2. LESA	SEAL, SALE		22. MWRA	WARM
3. TNLI	LINT		23. FRMI	FIRM
4. POSU	SOUP		24. MRET	TERM
5. LSIL	SILL		25. IDKS	DISK, KIDS, SKID
6. XYON	ONYX		26. EORB	BORE, ROBE
7. WTSE	STEW, WEST		27. SREO	ROSE, SORE
8. IFST	FIST, SIFT		28. NNEO	NEON, NONE
9. ELTF	FELT, LEFT		29. AILV	VIAL
10. ERLE	REEL, LEER		30. KEBA	BAKE, BEAK
11. RDCA	CARD		31. FLOD	FOLD
12. RCHA	ARCH, CHAR		32. RDAE	DEAR, READ, DARE
13. CDEI	DICE		33. ETPS	STEP, PETS
14. ERFA	FEAR		34. ERSU	SURE, RUSE
15. GIHS	SIGH		35. EILM	MILE, LIME
16. WKON	KNOW		36. IDOV	VOID
17. PLOO	LOOP, POOL, POLO		37. HEAC	EACH
18. ARWP	WRAP, WARP		38. ELNA	LANE, LEAN
19. WCEH	CHEW		39. AROR	ROAR
20. SAEV	SAVE, VASE		40. ITDE	DIET, TIED, TIDE

WORD LIST

5 LETTERS

1. REGEA	AGREE	
2. TRWAE	WATER	
3. SEILA	AISLE	
4. DLSEI	SLIDE	
5. SGTHO	GHOST	
6. OQTUE	QUOTE	
7. VEAHE	HEAVE	
8. GULAH	LAUGH	
9. ETUIQ	QUITE	
10. SREPA	PEARS, SPARE, SPEAR	
11. TRNOH	NORTH, THORN	
12. STAFE	FEAST	
13. SLAEE	EASEL, LEASE	
14. UTROE	OUTER, ROUTE	
15. GITSH	SIGHT	
16. MCHRA	MARCH, CHARM	
17. LISEM	SMILE, LIMES, MILES	
18. ECATH	TEACH, CHEAT	
19. TESEH	SHEET, THESE	
20. NKACS	SNACK	
21. WSRAE	SWEAR, WARES	
22. TIFUR	FRUIT	
23. CEPRI	PRICE	
24. EAPPR	PAPER	
25. DELIF	FIELD, FILED	
26. CTOIX	TOXIC	
27. LSLKI	SKILL, KILLS	
28. ENKEL	KNEEL	
29. KLENA	ANKLE	
30. HRCEO	CHORE	
31. TBAHE	BATHE	
32. DIOAR	RADIO	
33. RLWOD	WORLD	
34. ADLYI	DAILY	
35. NEOSI	NOISE	
36. RANBI	BRAIN	
37. LKBNA	BLANK	
38. WPORE	POWER	
39. RELNA	LEARN	
40. RSEPU	PURSE	

SUSTAINED ATTENTION TASK
ALPHABETIZING WORDS WITHIN SENTENCES

PURPOSE:

The purpose of this task is to improve the client's sustained attention for overall enhanced cognitive functioning.

DIRECTIONS:

Verbally present the client with sentences comprised of three to five words. Request that the client retain the sentence in short-term working memory and restate the words in alphabetical order.

TO INCREASE TASK DIFFICULTY:

1. Increase the length of the sentences.

2. Increase the content complexity of the sentences so they are more difficult to retain.

3. Increase the rate of stimulus presentation.

PRIMARY SKILLS TARGETED:

1. Sustained Attention

2. Alternating Attention

3. Working Memory Capacity and Efficiency

TO ADDRESS THE RELATED SKILL OF:	INCORPORATE THIS TASK MODIFICATION:
1. Speed of Processing	Impose time constraint (e.g., encourage client to restate words as quickly as possible)
2. Selective Attention	Complete task in a distracting environment (e.g., talk radio, others talking in background, visually distracting stimuli)

PERFORMANCE MEASURES:

Evaluate the following:

■ Ability to retain sentences in short-term memory long enough to alphabetize the words

■ Ability to alphabetize words in working memory

■ Percentage of words alphabetized correctly

■ Maximum number of words per sentence able to retain and alphabetize accurately

■ Length of time able to sustain attention to task before becoming fatigued

■ Effect of task modification(s) on performance (e.g., speed, distractions)

SENTENCES FOR WORD ALPHABETIZATION

3 WORDS

1. I feel good.	feel good I
2. Eat your dinner.	dinner Eat your
3. Open the door.	door Open the
4. Drink your tea.	Drink tea your
5. I was sick.	I sick was
6. Take the medicine.	medicine Take the
7. Call the doctor.	Call doctor the
8. May I go?	go I May
9. Where are they?	are they Where
10. We were late.	late We were
11. Wash your hands.	hands Wash your
12. Do not rush.	Do not rush
13. Are you warm?	Are warm you
14. She is mad.	is mad She
15. Bring the book.	book Bring the
16. Talk to me.	me Talk to
17. It is late.	is It late
18. Clean the kitchen.	Clean kitchen the
19. Do your work.	Do work your
20. Pass the pepper.	Pass pepper the
21. Knead the dough.	dough Knead the
22. Schedule the meeting.	meeting Schedule the
23. We went there.	there We went
24. You are funny.	are funny You
25. Do it soon.	Do it soon
26. Tom left town.	left Tom town
27. Laurie likes ballet.	ballet Laurie likes
28. They played basketball.	basketball played They
29. Save your money.	money Save your
30. Close your eyes.	Close eyes your
31. Give me that.	Give me that

Source: Adapted from C. Mateer and M. Moore-Sohlberg, (1992, September). *Current perspectives in cognitive rehabilitation.* Presented at conference entitled "Speaking of Cognition...Assessment and Intervention Strategies." Sponsored by Rehabilitation Services Midwest Medical Center: Indianapolis, IN. We appreciate their initial format idea, which stimulated the generation of our new sentence examples.

32. Cut the sandwich.	Cut sandwich the
33. Take me there.	me Take there
34. I am exhausted	am exhausted I
35. Time for breakfast.	breakfast for Time
36. Move it carefully.	carefully it Move
37. Make the bed.	bed Make the
38. Answer the telephone.	Answer telephone the
39. They went walking.	They walking went
40. Play the piano.	piano Play the
41. Lynn likes limes.	likes limes Lynn
42. He heard her.	He heard her
43. Is Isabelle in?	in Is Isabelle
44. Mary married Mark.	Mark married Mary
45. Tom took two.	Tom took two
46. She should shop.	She shop should
47. Debbie delegates duties.	Debbie delegates duties
48. They thought that.	that They thought
49. Kate knows Karen.	Karen Kate knows
50. Barbara brought bagels.	bagels Barbara brought

SENTENCES FOR ALPHABETIZATION

4 WORDS

1. Go to the store.	Go store the to
2. It is six o'clock.	is It o'clock six
3. Bring me the disks.	Bring disks me the
4. Where is the book?	book is the Where
5. Why aren't you here?	aren't here Why you
6. Thanksgiving is in November.	in is November Thanksgiving
7. May I borrow that?	borrow I May that
8. Where are we going?	are going we Where
9. How are you feeling?	are feeling How you
10. I found the dictionary.	dictionary found I the
11. I like orange juice.	I juice like orange
12. That baby looks happy.	baby happy looks That
13. When will you return?	return When will you
14. School was fun today.	fun School today was
15. I need to study.	I need study to
16. The radio doesn't work.	doesn't radio The work
17. What is on television?	is on television What
18. The movie was good.	good movie The was
19. You should be careful.	be careful should You
20. The comedian was hilarious.	comedian hilarious The was
21. I lost my ring.	I lost my ring
22. Make a dental appointment.	a appointment dental Make
23. Make a large donation.	a donation large Make
24. Did you see it?	Did it see you
25. Put the files away.	away files Put the
26. Take me with you.	me Take with you
27. Make a left turn.	a left Make turn
28. Follow the yellow signs.	Follow signs the yellow
29. I borrowed your car.	borrowed car I your
30. Anna really likes dogs.	Anna dogs likes really
31. Don't forget your vitamins.	Don't forget vitamins your

Source: Adapted from C. Mateer and M. Moore-Sohlberg, (1992, September). *Current perspectives in cognitive rehabilitation.* Presented at conference entitled "Speaking of Cognition...Assessment and Intervention Strategies." Sponsored by Rehabilitation Services Midwest Medical Center: Indianapolis, IN. We appreciate their initial format idea, which stimulated the generation of our new sentence examples.

32. The store is closed.   closed is store The

33. Alice became a doctor.   a Alice became doctor

34. I like your shoes.   I like shoes your

35. Who is coming over?   coming is over Who

36. She makes me smile.   makes me She smile

37. The law has changed.   changed has law The

38. Our office has moved.   has moved office Our

39. Winter is coming soon.   coming is soon Winter

40. She is getting big.   big getting is She

41. He hit his heel.   He heel his hit

42. Susie said she'd sue.   said she'd sue Susie

43. Danielle doesn't do dusting. Danielle do doesn't dusting

44. Brett bought blue blinds.   blinds blue bought Brett

45. We went walking Wednesday. walking We Wednesday went

46. Fred found four friends.   found four Fred friends

47. Matt made my meal.   made Matt meal my

48. Polly plays piano pieces.   piano pieces plays Polly

49. Leah loves licking lollipops. Leah licking lollipops loves

50. Ben bakes baked beans.   baked bakes beans Ben

SENTENCES FOR ALPHABETIZATION

5 WORDS

1. She was afraid of it.   afraid it of She was
2. Type it on the computer.   computer it on the Type
3. We need a new table.   a need new table We
4. You need your foot x-rayed.   foot need x-rayed You your
5. Your birthday is on Tuesday.   birthday is on Tuesday Your
6. Katie is going to college.   college going is Katie to
7. I like apples and apricots.   and apples apricots I like
8. He is a good friend.   a friend good He is
9. The dog came at me.   at came dog me The
10. Open my gift to you.   gift my Open to you
11. Send out the invitations today.   invitations out Send the today
12. Can you do it now?   Can do it now you
13. I don't understand your concern.   concern don't I understand your
14. Where did you find this?   did find this Where you
15. Who is your new friend?   friend is new Who your
16. I need two more dollars.   dollars I more need two
17. What is your favorite beverage?   beverage favorite is What your
18. I need to finish it.   finish I it need to
19. Chris has a good plan.   a Chris good has plan
20. Did they approve of it?   approve Did it of they
21. She will need a curfew.   a curfew need She will
22. The carpeting needs a cleaning.   a carpeting cleaning needs The
23. I wish we could go.   could go I we wish
24. I will apply for it.   apply for I it will
25. Can you call her tomorrow?   call Can her tomorrow you
26. The girls are having fun.   are fun girls having The
27. Where did we go wrong?   did go we Where wrong
28. There is a tornado watch.   a is There tornado watch
29. Did you make apple pie?   apple Did make pie you
30. He needs a new attitude.   a attitude He needs new
31. Be here by four o'clock.   Be by four here o'clock

Source: Adapted from C. Mateer and M. Moore-Sohlberg, (1992, September). *Current perspectives in cognitive rehabilitation.* Presented at conference entitled "Speaking of Cognition...Assessment and Intervention Strategies." Sponsored by Rehabilitation Services Midwest Medical Center: Indianapolis, IN. We appreciate their initial format idea, which stimulated the generation of our new sentence examples

32.	Tell me where to go.	go me Tell to where
33.	The ocean looks cold today.	cold looks ocean The today
34.	We really enjoyed our vacation.	enjoyed our really vacation We
35.	I have a bad cold.	a bad cold have I
36.	We have to meet soon.	have meet soon to We
37.	Should she finish it now?	finish it now she Should
38.	Your outfit looks too big.	big looks outfit too Your
39.	The birthday cake was delicious.	birthday cake delicious The was
40.	The interview went very well.	interview The very well went
41.	Michelle makes much more money.	makes Michelle money more much
42.	Why would Wayne want wreaths?	want Wayne Why would wreaths
43.	We were wrong weren't we?	We we were weren't wrong
44.	Sam said Sarah studies sociology.	said Sam Sarah sociology studies
45.	Sherri said Steve sells slippers.	said sells Sherri slippers Steve
46.	Tony talked to Tammy today.	talked Tammy to today Tony
47.	Donna did daring difficult deeds.	daring deeds did difficult Donna
48.	We won't walk will we?	walk we we will won't
49.	Emma eats eggs every evening.	eats eggs Emma evening every
50.	They thought that thing through.	that They thing thought through

SUSTAINED ATTENTION TASK
CALCULATING MONEY AMOUNTS

PURPOSE:

The purpose of this task is to improve the client's sustained attention for overall enhanced cognitive functioning.

DIRECTIONS:

Verbally present the client with several money amounts of increasing length and complexity and require him or her to retain the amounts in short-term working memory and calculate the sum without writing it down.

TO INCREASE TASK DIFFICULTY:

1. Increase the number of money amounts provided.

2. Present the coins in mixed order (see actual task).

3. Increase the rate of stimulus presentation.

PRIMARY SKILLS TARGETED:

1. Sustained Attention

2. Alternating Attention

3. Working Memory Capacity and Efficiency

TO ADDRESS THE RELATED SKILL OF: INCORPORATE THIS TASK MODIFICATION:

1. Speed of Processing — Impose time constraint (e.g., encourage client to calculate sums as quickly as possible)

2. Selective Attention — Complete task in a distracting environment (e.g., talk radio, others talking in background, visual distractions)

PERFORMANCE MEASURES:

Evaluate the following:

- Ability to retain money amounts in short-term memory long enough to calculate the sums

- Ability to calculate sums within working memory

- Percentage of sums calculated correctly

- Maximum number of amounts able to retain and calculate accurately

- Length of time able to sustain attention to task before becoming fatigued

- Effect of task modification(s) on performance (e.g., speed, distractions)

MONEY AMOUNTS

A. 2 Coins, Descending Order

1.	5 nickels, 3 pennies	$0.28
2.	2 dimes, 4 nickels	$0.40
3.	4 nickels, 9 pennies	$0.29
4.	3 half-dollars, 2 nickels	$1.60
5.	5 quarters, 3 pennies	$1.28
6.	5 half-dollars, 3 dimes	$2.80
7.	7 dimes, 8 pennies	$0.78
8.	1 quarter, 8 nickels	$0.65
9.	6 quarters, 3 dimes	$1.80
10.	4 dimes, 7 nickels	$0.75

B. 2 Coins, Ascending Order

1.	3 pennies, 8 nickels	$0.43
2.	2 pennies, 7 dimes	$0.72
3.	4 nickels, 6 dimes	$0.80
4.	2 dimes, 4 quarters	$1.20
5.	3 dimes, 3 half-dollars	$1.80
6.	6 pennies, 2 quarters	$0.56
7.	5 pennies, 6 half-dollars	$3.05
8.	8 nickels, 2 quarters	$0.90
9.	3 nickels, 4 half-dollars	$2.15
10.	3 quarters, 1 half-dollar	$1.25

C. 3 Coins, Descending Order

1.	3 dimes, 2 nickels, 1 penny	$0.41
2.	1 quarter, 2 dimes, 3 nickels	$0.60
3.	4 quarters, 1 dime, 2 pennies	$1.12
4.	2 half-dollars, 4 dimes, 1 nickel	$1.45
5.	3 half-dollars, 2 quarters, 6 nickels	$2.30
6.	4 quarters, 3 nickels, 8 pennies	$1.23
7.	2 half-dollars, 7 dimes, 9 pennies	$1.79
8.	4 half-dollars, 1 nickel, 6 pennies	$2.11
9.	3 quarters, 2 nickels, 5 pennies	$0.90
10.	1 half-dollar, 3 quarters, 7 pennies	$1.32

D. 3 Coins, Ascending Order

1.	3 pennies, 4 nickels, 2 dimes	$0.43
2.	2 dimes, 2 quarters, 2 half-dollars	$1.70
3.	6 pennies, 2 dimes, 2 quarters	$0.76
4.	3 nickels, 4 quarters, 2 half-dollars	$2.15
5.	8 pennies, 4 nickels, 2 half-dollars	$1.28
6.	2 pennies, 4 dimes, 4 half-dollars	$2.42
7.	3 nickels, 1 dime, 4 quarters	$1.25
8.	9 pennies, 7 nickels, 3 quarters	$1.19
9.	5 nickels, 2 dimes, 2 half-dollars	$1.45
10.	3 dimes, 2 quarters, 4 half-dollars	$2.80

E. 3 Coins, Mixed Order

1.	3 nickels, 2 pennies, 1 dime	$0.27
2.	1 dime, 2 half-dollars, 3 quarters	$1.85
3.	5 dimes, 6 pennies, 2 quarters	$1.06
4.	2 quarters, 3 nickels, 1 half-dollar	$1.15
5.	2 half-dollars, 6 pennies, 4 nickels	$1.26
6.	3 dimes, 4 half-dollars, 8 pennies	$2.38
7.	2 dimes, 4 nickels, 6 quarters	$1.90
8.	1 nickel, 2 pennies, 6 quarters	$1.57
9.	4 nickels, 3 half-dollars, 4 dimes	$2.10
10.	4 quarters, 8 dimes, 1 half-dollar	$2.30

F. 4 Coins, Descending Order

1.	4 quarters, 2 dimes, 3 nickels, 4 pennies	$1.39
2.	2 half-dollars, 2 quarters, 4 dimes, 2 nickels	$2.00
3.	1 half-dollar, 1 dime, 3 nickels, 8 pennies	$0.83
4.	3 half-dollars, 2 quarters, 4 nickels, 7 pennies	$2.27
5.	3 quarters, 3 dimes, 4 nickels, 8 pennies	$1.33
6.	1 half-dollar, 2 quarters, 3 dimes, 4 nickels	$1.50
7.	2 half-dollars, 6 dimes, 2 nickels, 6 pennies	$1.76
8.	4 half-dollars, 1 quarter, 5 nickels, 6 pennies	$2.56
9.	6 quarters, 2 dimes, 1 nickel, 3 pennies	$1.78
10.	5 half-dollars, 1 dime, 1 nickel, 5 pennies	$2.70

G. 4 Coins, Ascending Order

1. 2 pennies, 2 nickels, 2 dimes, 2 quarters $0.82
2. 4 nickels, 2 dimes, 1 quarter, 3 half-dollars $2.15
3. 2 pennies, 4 nickels, 2 dimes, 4 half-dollars $2.42
4. 3 pennies, 2 nickels, 1 quarter, 4 half-dollars $2.38
5. 1 penny, 3 nickels, 8 dimes, 2 quarters $1.46
6. 6 nickels, 1 dime, 2 quarters, 1 half-dollar $1.40
7. 5 pennies, 4 nickels, 5 dimes, 2 half-dollars $1.75
8. 4 pennies, 3 nickels, 2 quarters, 1 half-dollar $1.19
9. 2 pennies, 6 nickels, 3 dimes, 4 quarters $1.62
10. 3 pennies, 3 nickels, 4 dimes, 4 half-dollars $2.58

H. 4 Coins, Mixed Order

1. 2 quarters, 4 nickels, 3 pennies, 1 dime $0.83
2. 1 half-dollar, 3 dimes, 6 nickels, 4 quarters $2.10
3. 8 pennies, 4 half-dollars, 2 nickels, 4 dimes $2.58
4. 2 half-dollars, 3 pennies, 4 quarters, 2 nickels $2.13
5. 4 dimes, 6 quarters, 3 pennies, 1 nickel $1.98
6. 2 quarters, 1 half-dollar, 2 nickels, 6 pennies $1.16
7. 5 dimes, 2 half-dollars, 5 nickels, 2 pennies $1.77
8. 3 half-dollars, 2 nickels, 4 pennies, 1 quarter $1.89
9. 4 quarters, 3 pennies, 5 nickels, 2 dimes $1.48
10. 9 pennies, 6 nickels, 3 half-dollars, 1 dime $1.99

SUSTAINED ATTENTION TASK
WORD CREATION

PURPOSE:

The purpose of this task is to improve the client's ability to manipulate information retained in working memory to improve sustained attention and cognitive flexibility.

DIRECTIONS:

Verbally provide the client with a lengthy word and require the client to retain the word in working memory. Once held in working memory, instruct the client to create as many smaller words as possible from the larger word *without writing the stimulus word down on paper*. Ask the client to spell the initial word to ensure correct spelling.

INCREASE TASK DIFFICULTY:

1. Increase the number of letters per word to create from the larger word (e.g., accept only four- and five-letter words).

2. Increase the length and complexity of the provided word.

PRIMARY SKILLS TARGETED:

1. Sustained Attention
2. Cognitive Flexibility
3. Working Memory

TO ADDRESS THE RELATED SKILL OF:	INCORPORATE THIS TASK MODIFICATION:
1. Speed of Retrieval	Impose time constraint (e.g., create smaller words as quickly as possible after hearing larger word)
2. Selective Attention	Complete task in a distracting environment (e.g., talk radio, others talking in background, visual distractions)

PERFORMANCE MEASURES:

Evaluate the following:

- Average number of words created in predetermined time frame
- Average length of words created
- Ability to retain larger word in working memory
- Ability to manipulate letters of large word in working memory to create smaller words
- Effect of task modification(s) on performance (e.g., speed, distractions)

WORD CREATION

1. transportation
2. excitement
3. international
4. corporation
5. solutions
6. equitable
7. journey
8. publication
9. sensational
10. material
11. attention
12. article
13. conspiracy
14. television
15. university
16. accidental
17. confusion
18. metropolitan
19. aviation
20. structure
21. decoration
22. instrumental
23. powerless
24. remembrance
25. united
26. telephone
27. representative
28. informative
29. delegation
30. agitation
31. literature
32. occupation
33. snowmobile
34. pyramid
35. fundamental
36. programmer
37. assistance
38. treatment
39. principal
40. coordination

SELECTIVE ATTENTION TASK
DISTRACTIONS TO UTILIZE WITH SUSTAINED ATTENTION TASKS

By utilizing these distractions while administering the previous sustained attention tasks or others you have created, you will be addressing selective attention.

- Turn on talk radio or televised news while providing task instructions or as the client is completing a task.

- Have the client face a window as a visual distraction.

- Choose a room close to a busy hallway and leave the door open.

- Occasionally turn the lights off or on.

- Talk with another person while the client is working on a task.

- Tap the table with a pen while directions are being provided and followed.

- Drop paper or a pen just as the client begins to follow directions.

- Make distracting noises such as turning the pages of a book, writing with a pencil, typing on the computer, talking to self aloud, tearing paper, whispering.

- Have other people intermittently come into the room.

- Sit in a room with a telephone and instruct the client to answer it when it rings (prior to the therapy session, instruct the secretary or a colleague to call the room and ask for you).

- Turn on a timer, that the client can hear, while completing an attention task that has a speed requirement.

ALTERNATING ATTENTION TASK
NAME AND COMPANY SORTING

PURPOSE:

The purpose of this task is to improve the client's ability to readily alternate his or her attention between written stimuli when verbally cued.

DIRECTIONS:

Provide the client with index cards with company and employee names (samples included to cut and paste on index cards). Instruct the client to alphabetize by company name and place cards in a single stack on the left. Instruct the client to "switch" when verbally cued and begin alphabetizing by employee's last name, placing those cards in a single stack on the right. Continue to have the client alternate alphabetizing by company and employee names by randomly interrupting the client and telling him or her to "switch." *Clinician must pay close attention to document that client appropriately alternates when cued, between company and employee names.* Periodically ask the client whether he or she is sorting by company or employee name to determine accuracy when compared to clinician's tally.

TO INCREASE TASK DIFFICULTY:

1. Increase the number of index cards to sort.
2. Increase the speed and number of times cued to "switch."

PRIMARY SKILLS TARGETED:

1. Alternating Attention
2. Sustained Attention

TO ADDRESS THE RELATED SKILL OF:	INCORPORATE THIS TASK MODIFICATION:
1. Speed of Processing	Impose time constraint (must complete alphabetizing of cards within specified time)
2. Selective Attention	Complete task in a distracting environment (e.g., news talk radio, others talking in background, visual distractions)

PERFORMANCE MEASURES:

Evaluate the following:

■ Transition time required to alternate between tasks (i.e., resumes alphabetizing after told to switch with or without difficulty)

■ Ability to organize information efficiently and accurately

■ The need for repetition of instructions or verbal cue to "switch"

■ Ability to independently utilize compensatory strategies while sorting

■ Effect of task modification(s) on performance (e.g., speed, distractions)

SAMPLE NAMES TO SORT

Thermopane Window Repair
ATTN: Luke Lancaster
6834 Chelsea Road
Boise, Idaho

American Appliance
ATTN: Sam Thompson
7084 Schoolcraft
Queens, New York

Materials Manufacturing
ATTN: Eric Woolfovitch
6625 Capitol Drive
Bridgewater, Massachusetts

Wheaton Construction Co.
ATTN: David Dorian
9882 North River Drive
Wheaton, Ohio

Information Systems Consultants
ATTN: Beth Elias
30301 Orchard Lake Road
Birmingham, Alabama

McDonald Excavating
ATTN: Patrick McDonald
5086 Northwestern Hwy
Allen Park, Georgia

Appraising and Antiques
ATTN: Paulette Gerard
6626 Hamilton Road
South Bend, Indiana

Sterling Jewelry Sales
ATTN: Anita Sommerville
2112 Whitewater Avenue
Seattle, Washington

Universal Plumbing
ATTN: Don Hammond
29068 Riverside Drive
White Plains, New York

Lighting Designs, Inc.
ATTN: Victoria Davis
836 Pinetree Circle
Sandusky, Ohio

Five Star Electronics
ATTN: Jack Brooks
120 Mack Avenue
Manhattan, New York

Chiropractic Consultants
ATTN: Brad Jacobson
14104 Civic Center Drive
Nashville, Tennessee

University Book Store
ATTN: Sarah Rothman
5515 Grove Street West
East Lansing, Michigan

Fine Furniture Repair
ATTN: Arnold Johnson
7654 State Street
Northfield, Minnesota

Security Systems, Inc.
ATTN: Joseph White
31300 Telegraph Road
Cleveland, Ohio

Investment Management
ATTN: Robert Curry
18510 Woodward Avenue
Greenfield, Pennsylvania

Rainforest Irrigation Systems
ATTN: Gary Gustav
2608 Liberty Road
San Jose, California

Incredible Ice Cream Treats
ATTN: Susan Landers
4243 Michigan Avenue
Naples, Florida

Sun Graphics Studio
ATTN: Maryann Baker
1036 Centerline Road
Scottsdale, Arizona

Environmental Engineers
ATTN: Raymond Cousins
557 Oakley Boulevard
Los Angeles, California

Bates Fishing Gear
ATTN: Mark Bates
2200 Piermont Avenue
Lake Lansing, Michigan

Equitable Solutions
ATTN: Joseph Stuben
6631 Doorshire Drive
Bangor, Maine

Computer Services Consultants
ATTN: Jeffrey Atkins
12543 Holmington
Jackson, Wyoming

N & H Hardware
ATTN: Harold Zeman
2122 Michigan Avenue
Chicago, Illinois

Futuristic Flowers
ATTN: Rose McDonald
3123 Bud Lane
Honolulu, Hawaii

Havenworth Hotel
ATTN: Gloria Stein
92387 Atwater Circle
Syracuse, New York

Paramount Pet Photographers
ATTN: Debbie Thomas
40998 Chimney Drive
Tampa, Florida

Nancy's Nail Design
ATTN: Nancy Ford
775 Davidson Drive
Madison, Wisconsin

Downtown Dental Services
ATTN: David York
117 Center Street
Santa Rosa, California

Selective Tires
ATTN: Molly Sawyer
4567 Cactus Court
San Antonio, Texas

Thomas Tees and Things
ATTN: Joshua Andrews
21648 Blue Skies Street
Denver, Colorado

Centurian Motors
ATTN: Samuel Morris
12432 Atwolden Court
Buffalo, New York

Travel To Go
ATTN: Juli Goodfellow
43112 Sheldon Court
Mansfield, Illinois

Spectrum Landscaping
ATTN: Meghan Fudge
19699 Ironwood Drive
Plymouth, Maryland

Advanced Solutions
ATTN: Marvin Waters
7567 Jefferson
Charleston, Virginia

Management Affairs
ATTN: Martha Stevens
515 Professional Court
Columbus, Ohio

Community Health Spa
ATTN: Barbara Billings
9087 Liberty
Denver, Colorado

Knight Protection Services
ATTN: Kenneth Knight
90800 Main Street
Pittsburg, Pennsylvania

Allied Appliances
ATTN: Karen Circuit
9090 Welch Road
Albuquerque, New Mexico

Treetop Trimming Services
ATTN: Larry Meyers
22446 Pinecroft
Eugene, Oregon

Grady's Convenience Store
ATTN: Steven Grady
14533 Meadowbrook Lane
Myrtle Beach, South Carolina

Quality Tuxedo Rentals
ATTN: Todd Jackson
567 First Street
Fargo, Minnesota

Unique Toys and Gifts
ATTN: Kathy White
900 Peters Lane
Blaine, Washington

National Blueprint
ATTN: Elaine Pauly
223 Vaughan Road
Hibbing, Minnesota

Gold Star Jewelry
ATTN: Vic Little
390 Adams Lane
Memphis, Tennessee

Mattress Galleries
ATTN: Alex Jones
9800 Palmer Road
Richfield, Utah

Guaranteed Mortgage
ATTN: David Fisher
41232 Fox Street
Anchorage, Alaska

Fred's Furniture Repair
ATTN: Fred Firestone
39000 Rivard Drive
Dover, Delaware

Westland Funeral Home
ATTN: Mort Sanford
617 Grand Avenue
Westland, New York

Altitude Aviation
ATTN: Alan Stevens
3479 Old Blanco Road
Carmel, California

Quick Subs & Sandwiches
ATTN: Mike Conner
55600 Telegraph Road
Seattle, Washington

Village Realtors
ATTN: Susan Moore
7782 James Boulevard
Hershey, Pennsylvania

Behavioral Hotline
ATTN: Larry Chance
4001 Greentree Road
Chicago, Illinois

Concord Cleaners
ATTN: Paul Curtis
11345 Deerfield
Toronto, Canada

The Golden River
ATTN: Greg Meadows
4222 Victory Circle
Redford, Michigan

Imagine You Salon
ATTN: Sandy King
1778 River Road
Tempe, Arizona

The Cutting Edge
ATTN: Erica Crain
900 Eureka Boulevard
Hollywood, California

Classic Comic Company
ATTN: Jeffrey Fink
877 Conant Street
Annapolis, Maryland

Chuck's Clippers
ATTN: Chuck Smith
5788 Town Drive
Roosevelt, Utah

Kids Corner Daycare
ATTN: Diane Cooper
8771 Stuart Drive
Springfield, Illinois

ALTERNATING ATTENTION TASK
VERBAL INTERRUPTIONS WHILE READING

PURPOSE:

The purpose of this task is to improve the client's ability to readily alternate his or her attention between a written and verbal stimulus.

DIRECTIONS:

Provide the client with a lengthy reading passage of personal relevance and ask that he or she read the article for later discussion. While reading, randomly interrupt the client and verbally provide instructions for the client to write down for later recall (have the client create a note-taking sheet or utilize the Cue Sheet provided in this chapter). On completion of the task, ask the client to discuss the article to ensure comprehension. Additionally, review the list of instructions written down by the client to ensure accurate processing and recording of the information.

TO INCREASE TASK DIFFICULTY:

1. Increase the complexity of the reading passage.
2. Increase the length and detail of each instruction.
3. Increase the speed of presentation of each instruction.

PRIMARY SKILLS TARGETED:

1. Alternating Attention
2. Sustained Attention
3. Verbal Information Processing
4. Written Information Processing

TO ADDRESS THE RELATED SKILL OF: INCORPORATE THIS TASK MODIFICATION:

TO ADDRESS THE RELATED SKILL OF:	INCORPORATE THIS TASK MODIFICATION:
1. Speed of Processing	Impose time constraint (e.g., read passage within a specific amount of time)
2. Selective Attention	Complete task in a distracting environment (e.g., talk radio, others talking in background, visual distractions)

PERFORMANCE MEASURES:

Evaluate the following:

■ Transition time required to alternate between tasks (i.e., resumes reading with or without difficulty)

■ Ability to accurately record important information efficiently and thoroughly

■ The need for repetition of informational segments

- Ability to independently utilize compensatory strategies while reading, such as marking where stopped reading or making notes in the margin

- Percentage of instructions encoded and recorded accurately (allow to refer to notes)

- Percentage of reading comprehension questions responded to accurately

- Effect of task modification(s) on performance (e.g., speed, distractions)

LIST OF INSTRUCTIONS FOR INTERRUPTING READING

You may wish to modify these instructions according to a specific job interest for a given client.

1. Jan will see you tonight at 7:00.

2. The preliminary sketches for the perfume bottle design are due on Mr. Edward's desk tomorrow at 8:00 a.m.

3. You'll need DeskTop Publishing for the Life Magazine project.

4. Your secretary needs your billing sheet by the end of the day today.

5. Nathan needs a ride home today at 5:30.

6. Annette Fields needs to meet you regarding the Fletcher account at 7:00 a.m. on Thursday.

7. Todd would like to meet for lunch today at 1:15 at the Olive Garden Restaurant. Please call to confirm.

8. Call Anita when you get a chance.

9. Your doctor called to reschedule your appointment for Friday at 2:00 p.m. Please call to confirm.

10. Call in an order for the new graphics program *Grapharts*.

11. Meet Terri Murry at 3:00 p.m. in the conference room.

12. Touch base with Marci about the company picnic.

13. Calculate an estimate for the Penfield Contract.

14. John Merle needs the project on his desk by 6:00 p.m.—give it to his assistant Kristine.

15. Avis is collecting $20.00 from everyone for a gift for Beth. She needs it by next week.

16. Call Ms. Wellstone about the advertising slogan for the Bergman contract.

17. There will be a meeting this morning in conference room B at 10:00 a.m. Bring your ideas for the new training manual.

18. Finish loading the two new graphics programs onto your computer.

19. Every Monday give Vicki an estimate of your hours billed each week.

20. See Paul Hammou sometime today.

21. Call Pam Spigarelli regarding the Computer Novelties contract.

22. Tell Ricky and David about the staff meeting being changed from Thursday to Friday.

23. We will be closing early on the 23rd.

24. Gregory needs a copy of the mailing list.

25. Bernadette needs a decision by next Monday on which sales manuals we should purchase.

26. You have a meeting with Mr. Vincent and Ms. Stockton on Wednesday at 1:00 p.m. Bring your budget analysis.

27. Mr. Bonner from Q-Tech would like to discuss the estimate with you.

28. Ms. Rennie from Accounting needs to discuss your 1997 cost analysis. Please call her at extension 256.

29. Check your house mail for the confidential document regarding your pay.

30. Leave a message on Richard Brown's voice mail regarding your proposed deadline for completion of the data-base program on which you are working. The number is (613) 465-3043, extension 2489.

31. When you have an opportunity today, please page Judy at (204) 564-3985. She needs your expertise to answer a client's question.

32. You will need to assign a sales agent to the Hank's account.

33. Be sure to send Tricia Preston a copy of the contract for the logo design before the 30th of this month. Her address is Raydon Materials, 3409 Lancaster, Richmond, Louisiana 46568.

34. Russ from Personnel returned your call. He'll be in until 3:00 p.m.

35. Linda called to ask your advice about the upcoming presentation.

36. Call Dan before 4:00 p.m., but after 1:00 p.m.

37. Phyllis can meet for lunch either Thursday at 12:30 or Friday at 1:30.

38. Call Andrew tomorrow at (616) 238-4199, extension 605.

39. You are scheduled to speak next Wednesday from 10:00 to 12:00.

CUE SHEET FOR WRITING DOWN INSTRUCTIONS

THINGS TO DO:

1.   6.

2.   7.

3.   8.

4.   9.

5.   10.

CALLS TO MAKE:

1.   6.

2.   7.

3.   8.

4.   9.

5.   10.

PEOPLE TO SEE:

1.   6.

2.   7.

3.   8.

4.   9.

5.   10.

ALTERNATING ATTENTION TASK
MOTOR AND COGNITIVE TASK IDEAS

DIRECTIONS:

To address alternating attention, select either two motor tasks or two cognitive tasks listed below and require the client to alternate between each of the two tasks, switching attentional focus whenever randomly indicated by the clinician.

MOTOR TASKS

- Separate deck of cards into suits, numbers, or colors
- Separate deck of cards into piles of even or odd numbers
- Sort coins
- Sort small objects (e.g., paper clips, nuts, bolts)
- Put papers in numerical order
- Sort large and small paper clips
- Sort colored index cards
- Organize magazines by month
- Put pictures in a photo album
- Separate coupons according to expired and unexpired dates
- Sort colored rubber bands
- Separate new and used file folders

COGNITIVE TASKS

- Respond to yes/no questions
- Respond to thought-provoking questions
- Engage in a conversation
- Talk on the telephone
- Solve math problems in working memory
- Determine if two presented sentences have the same meaning
- Generate items in requested categories
- Provide definitions for specific words
- Provide synonyms or antonyms for specific words
- Put a target word into a sentence
- Unscramble words
- Determine if sentences make sense

DIVIDED ATTENTION TASK
PROCESSING LETTERS WHILE SORTING CARDS

PURPOSE:

The purpose of this task is to improve the client's ability to divide his or her attention between two different stimuli, in order to complete both a cognitive and motor task simultaneously.

DIRECTIONS:

Instruct the client to separate a deck of cards by suit, while simultaneously listening to a verbal presentation of four letters that spell a word. The client must verbally provide the word being spelled while continuing to sort cards.

TO INCREASE TASK DIFFICULTY:

1. Increase the length of stimulus word provided to five or six letters.
2. Request a faster pace for card sorting.
3. Present letters at a faster pace.

PRIMARY SKILLS TARGETED:

1. Divided Attention
2. Alternating Attention
3. Sustained Attention

TO ADDRESS THE RELATED SKILL OF:

INCORPORATE THIS TASK MODIFICATION:

1. Speed of Processing — Impose time constraint when determining word being spelled

2. Selective Attention — Complete task in a distracting environment (e.g., talk radio, others talking in background, visual distractions)

PERFORMANCE MEASURES:

Evaluate the following:

- Percentage of words determined correctly
- Percentage of cards sorted correctly
- Ability to execute both tasks simultaneously
- Total time required to complete a certain number of words
- Effect of task modification(s) on performance (e.g., speed, distractions)

WORD LIST

4 LETTERS

1. hall	real	belt	deer	fame
2. jail	goal	chip	bird	hike
3. wall	hurt	gown	coal	bake
4. will	bark	sift	boot	deep
5. self	cave	fail	ache	slap
6. camp	glue	bowl	coin	slid
7. pole	farm	like	yell	life
8. brag	milk	file	cord	talk
9. sale	bran	down	foul	soul
10. pile	sail	bald	mail	June
11. pain	look	tank	hair	seat
12. room	feel	bath	lion	beat
13. gate	sill	gram	ring	vein
14. dish	give	save	roll	come
15. fall	feet	worm	felt	link
16. sell	keep	talk	high	draw
17. sort	gaze	sand	slim	joke
18. salt	know	tent	love	late
19. work	play	nine	five	thin
20. fork	four	sign	nail	plot
21. pill	doll	spin	gasp	grip
22. zone	veal	zest	weak	free
23. snow	ears	play	ploy	pray
24. prod	stew	goat	gray	glow
25. oust	quit	know	kite	jeep
26. dime	home	bush	copy	they
27. bike	heel	join	lift	vine
28. hang	lace	true	chin	lend
29. seal	dock	flow	fool	mile
30. lock	game	film	soil	food
31. have	fist	more	lime	door
32. soot	rule	wine	gold	neck
33. band	your	warm	mice	pack
34. bait	cone	lied	bank	task

35. fend   baby   wing   slip   brag

36. book   wear   hire   turn   plan

37. bear   stem   eyes   sewn   plea

38. tint   beak   soon   aunt   rack

39. tape   rain   fuse   plug   dust

40. wire   cane   punt   sigh   oven

DIVIDED ATTENTION TASK

ATTENDING TO MULTIPLE STIMULI WHILE SCANNING PARAGRAPHS

PURPOSE:

The purpose of this task is to improve the client's ability to attend to multiple stimuli simultaneously for enhanced divided attention skills.

DIRECTIONS:

Provide the client with a page of typed information (from a book or magazine) and the following directions written at the top of the page:

1. Circle all "the's"

2. Cross out all commas with an "x"

3. Cross out all capital letters with a slash

Request the client to scan the information rather than reading for content and execute all three directions at once.

TO INCREASE TASK DIFFICULTY:

1. Increase the number or complexity of commands to be followed.

2. Increase the length of the typed information so that the client must divide his or her attention for a longer period of time.

3. Request a faster pace for task completion.

4. Ask basic content questions related to the information.

PRIMARY SKILLS TARGETED:

1. Divided Attention

2. Alternating Attention

3. Sustained Attention

4. Attention to Details

TO ADDRESS THE RELATED SKILL OF:	INCORPORATE THIS TASK MODIFICATION:
1. Speed of Processing	Impose time constraint to complete scanning and execution of directions
2. Selective Attention	Complete task in a distracting environment (e.g., talk radio, others talking in background, visual distractions)

PERFORMANCE MEASURES:

Evaluate the following:

■ Percentage of targets correctly located

■ Percentage of targets having correct marking

■ Percentage of errors self-corrected when cued to review page again

■ Time required to complete task

■ Effect of task modification(s) on performance (e.g., speed, distractions)

DIVIDED ATTENTION TASK
MOTOR AND COGNITIVE TASK IDEAS

DIRECTIONS:

To address divided attention, select one motor task and one cognitive task from the lists below and require the client to engage in both tasks simultaneously.

MOTOR TASKS

■ Separate deck of cards into suits, numbers, or colors

■ Separate deck of cards into piles of even or odd numbers

■ Sort coins by amount

■ Sort small objects (e.g., paper clips, nuts, bolts)

■ Put papers in numerical order

■ Sort large and small paper clips

■ Sort colored index cards

■ Organize magazines by month

■ Put pictures in a photo album

■ Separate coupons according to expired and unexpired dates

■ Sort colored rubber bands

■ Separate new and used file folders

COGNITIVE TASKS

■ Respond to yes/no questions

■ Respond to thought-provoking questions

■ Engage in a conversation

■ Talk on the telephone

■ Solve math problems in working memory

■ Determine if two presented sentences have the same meaning

■ Generate items in requested categories

■ Provide definitions for specific words

■ Provide synonyms or antonyms for specific words

■ Put a target word into a sentence

■ Unscramble words

■ Determine if sentences make sense

HOME PRACTICE TASKS

Several of the ideas listed below can be completed during the monitoring period of treatment, with the therapist recording client performance. Other ideas may be suggested to the client upon discharge to promote maintenance of therapy gains.

■ Force yourself to concentrate for gradually increasing periods of time (use a timer or watch to track the time)

■ Practice attention strategies to sustain your attention during movies and leisure reading

■ Add increasing levels of distractions while reading or listening, to build up your tolerance for noise

■ Alternate between two tasks (e.g., reading the newspaper and making cookies or paying household bills and doing the laundry)

■ Attempt to complete a physical and mental task simultaneously (e.g., fold laundry while talking on the telephone)

■ If able to concentrate, attempt to have television or news talk radio playing while you are completing tasks around the house (e.g., cleaning, laundry, paying bills, making telephone calls)

SUGGESTIONS FOR FAMILIES

■ Limit as many distractions as possible in the home environment when requesting family member to listen or follow instructions

■ Allow family member to finish concentrating on what he or she may be doing prior to interrupting with something new or different

■ Be certain that your family member is visibly paying attention when speaking to him or her

■ Allow time for family member to "switch gears" when changing tasks or topics

■ Expect the need for breaks due to mental fatigue

■ Encourage family member to stop other tasks when attempting to discuss a topic or listen to others' comments or instructions

■ If family member appears to have forgotten, consider that he or she may have not heard you in the first place due to difficulty with paying attention

■ Provide verbal cues when necessary, such as "Did you hear all of that? Are you focusing on what I am saying?"

■ Inquire about therapy, skills areas addressed, and improvements

■ Inquire about compensatory strategies used and which work best; attempt to monitor your family member's use of strategies

CHAPTER 5

Treating Functional and Prospective Memory Impairments

DEFINITIONS

Functional Memory

A cognitive-language skill that relies on the abilities of perception, attention, encoding, storage, and retrieval of specific information and is required for new learning, information recall, and daily functioning. Difficulties with attention may lead to inaccurate encoding and storage and unsuccessful retrieval of verbal and written information. Impairments in encoding or storage may result in limited integration of new information with previous knowledge and decreased comprehension of information. Lastly, difficulties with retrieval may result in a reduced ability to access stored information for future recall and use.

Prospective Memory

With respect to prospective memory, Winograd (1988) states: "There can hardly be a more practical aspect of memory than remembering to do things at the appropriate time" (p. 348). This ability is necessary for the completion of such daily tasks as taking medication, returning a telephone call, and keeping an appointment.

Specific to the mild-to-moderate TBI population, impairments in these skill areas may manifest themselves in difficulties such as:

- Reduced encoding secondary to an attention or information-processing difficulty, not a perceptual problem

- Inefficient storage due to limitations in organization skills and working memory capacity

- Reduced retrieval of information

- Reduced recall of tasks to complete at specific times

- Limitations in follow-through for both verbal and nonverbal daily memory demands

- Difficulty with consistently remembering to utilize learned compensatory strategies for any skill limitations

OTHER CONTRIBUTING COGNITIVE IMPAIRMENTS

The following are cognitive impairments that may be seen in people with mild-to-moderate TBI which may exacerbate a functional **memory** impairment:

Difficulties with:	May lead to:
1. Attention/Concentration	Difficulty sustaining attention to accurately encode, store, and retrieve information (sustained attention)
	Difficulty shifting focus to accurately encode, store, and retrieve information (alternating attention)
	Difficulty sustaining attention in the presence of distractions to accurately encode, store, and retrieve information (selective attention)

2. Organization   Disorganized storage of information resulting in retrieval difficulties

Reduced integration of new information with previous knowledge resulting in retention difficulties

3. Speed of Processing   Delayed processing of information, causing one to miss important facts or details

4. Executive Functioning   Reduced ability to initiate use of suggested compensatory memory strategies

Decreased ability to self-monitor use of suggested compensatory memory strategies

The following are cognitive impairments that may be seen in people with mild-to-moderate TBI that may exacerbate a **prospective memory** impairment:

Difficulties with: **May lead to:**

1. Attention   Becoming distracted and forgetting what task needs to be completed at a specified time

2. Organization   Ineffective or inconsistent implementation of compensatory memory strategies to assist in recall of tasks and responsibilities to be completed

3. Executive Functioning   Decreased ability to plan when tasks and activities need to be scheduled or completed

Reduced initiation to utilize suggested compensatory memory strategies

Reduced time sense, which interferes with timely completion of tasks

FUNCTIONAL IMPLICATIONS OF MEMORY IMPAIRMENTS

The following is a list of many of the abilities needed for successful communication in the natural environments of home, work, and school. Impairments in functional and prospective memory in people with mild-to-moderate TBI may present communication concerns that compromise performance in these functional environments. You are encouraged to explore these and other related activities with your clients to create functional and personally relevant therapy tasks and to maximize carryover of therapeutic gains to the natural environment.

Functional Memory

In the Home

Ability to...

■ Effectively encode, store, and retrieve information for independent daily living

Examples:

Retain and recall radio and television reports

Recall verbal information provided by others

Retain and recall information from magazine and newspaper articles

Recall information needed to resolve problems or make decisions

At Work

Ability to...

■ Effectively encode, store, and retrieve information for job task completion and effectiveness

Examples:

Recall complex or lengthy information

Remember responses to your questions asked of supervisor or coworkers

Retain newly learned information from meetings

Retain newly learned information from memos, manuals, or other written correspondence

At School

Ability to...

■ Effectively encode, store, and retrieve information for academic success

Examples:

Recall verbal information from lectures

Recall written information from textbooks

Retrieve learned information to successfully complete quizzes and examinations

Recall complex or lengthy information to solve problems

Complete oral examinations successfully

Respond to questions regarding reading assignments

Explain homework requirements

Participate in classroom discussions

Prospective Memory (attention, planning, initiation, and self-monitoring)

In the Home

Ability to...

■ Effectively remember to do things in the future at a specified time

Examples:

Schedule appointments

Make and return personal telephone calls

Mail birthday and holiday cards

Set personal alarm clock to allow adequate preparation time

Take medication as directed

Recall specific items when shopping

At Work

Ability to...

■ Effectively remember to do things in the future at designated times

Examples:

Attend staff meetings

Attend professional conferences

Make and return business telephone calls

Provide telephone messages to colleagues

Relay accurate information to others on time

At School

Ability to...

■ Effectively remember to do things in the future to meet academic demands

Examples:

Attend scheduled school events

Attend planned club meetings

Attend sporting events

Complete homework assignments in a timely manner

Attend to test dates and incorporate preparation time into study schedule

In addition to the memory tasks provided in the following pages, you may utilize the information listed above to create unique therapy tasks that will be most meaningful for your client, depending upon his or her goal environment. Please refer to the cover sheet for each task to assist you in addressing related skills simultaneously.

COMPENSATORY STRATEGIES

Select from this list the memory strategies that would be most assistive to your clients and effectively utilized by them, considering their skill limitations and potential home, work, and school environments. It is recommended that these strategies be taught to the client and incorporated into the therapy sessions until the client is able to utilize them successfully and independently. Additionally, allow for practice of the specific strategy in the target environment to ensure successful carryover.

Encoding

- Silently tell yourself "pay attention" while listening and reading

- Minimize distractions in your environment to assist with accurate encoding of information

- Repeat information aloud to ensure accurate encoding of information

- Whenever possible, encode information through multiple modalities (i.e., read, listen, view).

- Whenever possible, utilize your strongest processing modality when encoding information

Storage and Integration

- Use self-questions, as understanding enhances memory (e.g., "Do I understand? Do I need to ask a question? How is this meaningful to me? How does this fit with what I know?")

- Paraphrase and summarize incoming information into your own words

- Scan for and impose some order on incoming information (e.g., outline or use note cards) and practice output as organization occurs at output, as well as input

- Use diagrams or forms to organize information. This will facilitate deeper encoding and integration of information, and its subsequent retrieval

- Relate the incoming information to personal life experiences and current knowledge

- Visualize verbal information in graphs, pictures, cartoons, or action-based imagery (e.g., picture yourself carrying out the action). Begin with concrete images (e.g., cup, pen) and then move to abstract actions and emotions (e.g., washing, angry)

- Group items into "chunks" (e.g., telephone numbers)

- Categorize by similarities or differences

Retrieval

- Use mnemonics (i.e., letter or word to recall specific information)

- Use key and cue words to stimulate retrieval of important main ideas and details

- Use semantic knowledge of basic scripts (e.g., picture yourself in a discussion or situation) to help reconstruct previous events and recall related information

■ Refer to outline or notecards of organized information

■ Use self-questions to prompt recall of information

■ Utilize created images to recall related information

Functional Memory

■ Use external memory aids such as:

a journal

written notes

a calendar

checklists

written or pictured time lines

Post-it™ notes

■ Use electronic devices such as:

pagers

telephone dialers (preprogrammed numbers or redial button)

voice-activated telephone dialing

calculators

car finders

tape recorders

key finders

answering machines

a laptop computer

■ Rehearse information

■ Relate information to personal life experiences and current knowledge

■ During retrieval, reconstruct the environment in which information was received

■ Keep items (e.g., purse, car keys) in designated places and recall through use of visual imagery

■ To recall names:

a. Have person repeat name as you say it aloud

b. Establish an association with someone famous or someone you know

c. Repeat the name to yourself several times and visualize the person's face or exaggerate a special feature

d. Use the person's name aloud during conversation

FUNCTIONAL MEMORY TASK

ERRAND RECALL

PURPOSE:

The purpose of this task is to improve the client's ability to recall errands following a time delay and distraction to improve functional memory skills.

DIRECTIONS:

Present the client with three hypothetical errands to remember. Instruct the client to remember the errands for later recall. To provide a time delay and distraction, verbally present a thought-provoking question to the client. After answering the clinician's question, request the client to recall the three errands.

TO INCREASE TASK DIFFICULTY:

1. Increase the number of errands presented for recall.
2. Increase complexity of errands to recall (e.g., add details such as color, number of objects, specific locations, designated times).
3. Ask more than one thought-provoking question to increase the time delay and level of distraction before recalling the errands.
4. Increase the rate of presentation of errands.

PRIMARY SKILLS TARGETED:

1. Encoding of Information
2. Storage of Information
3. Delayed Retrieval of Information
4. Sustained Attention
5. Alternating Attention

TO ADDRESS THE RELATED SKILL OF:	INCORPORATE THIS TASK MODIFICATION:
1. Speed of Retrieval	Impose time constraint (e.g., recall errands as quickly as possible after answering question)
2. Selective Attention	Complete task in a distracting environment (e.g., talk radio, others talking in background)

PERFORMANCE MEASURES:

Evaluate the following:

■ Average number of presented errands retained and recalled accurately following a time delay and distraction

■ Ability to recall specific details pertaining to errand

■ Ability to generate an appropriate answer to a thought-provoking question

■ Effect of task modification(s) on performance (e.g., speed, distractions, change in focus)

ERRANDS FOR RECALL

1. Turn off coffee
2. Take stereo in for repair
3. Return eyeglasses for repair
Q: What do you do to relax after a stressful event or day?

1. Pick up neighbor's mail
2. Return red blouse
3. Wash new black pants
Q: What do you think about that brings a smile to your face?

1. Take winter sweaters to dry cleaners
2. Take brown shoes in for repair
3. Clean the basement window screens
Q: What is an activity that you most enjoy doing with family or friends and why?

1. Change dentist appointment to next Friday
2. Ask your friend to dinner on Saturday
3. Call your mother tonight at 5:30 p.m.
Q: What are you able to do well that makes you proud of yourself?

1. Confirm savings bonds amounts
2. Deposit check
3. Return two library books
Q: Why is it important to stay informed about current events?

1. Turn on lawn sprinklers
2. Pick out birthday cards for nephew and sister
3. Schedule hair cut for next Tuesday
Q: What is a promise that you would like to make to yourself and keep?

1. Take paper and aluminum cans to recycling center
2. Pick up a video on a place you would like to visit
3. Pick up a gallon of chocolate yogurt
Q: What is something you have a hard time forgiving?

1. Take broken necklace to jeweler to fix clasp
2. Get gas for the lawnmower and edger
3. Weed front and back flower beds

Q: What qualities do you most respect in other people?

1. Wash and wax car
2. Cut out coupons from Sunday paper
3. Return shirt you received for your birthday

Q: What is something that recently happened that restored your faith in people?

1. Pick up more dog food
2. Drop off film for developing
3. Pack up household trash for pick-up

Q: Where have you spent five good days in a row?

1. Shop for brother's birthday gift
2. Call sister for aunt's address
3. Order pizza for dinner and make a salad
4. Cancel doctor appointment

Q: What are you looking forward to next month?

1. Go to travel agent to pick up vacation information
2. Withdraw $40 from automatic teller machine or bank
3. Buy a book of stamps from the post office
4. Inquire about piano lessons

Q: What are two things that you like about yourself?

1. Buy wrapping paper for shower gift
2. Go to bank to inquire about a loan
3. Call cable company regarding poor cable reception
4. Find out your new bank's hours

Q: What is a recent personal accomplishment?

1. Take car in for oil change
2. Call for tickets to hockey game
3. Buy vacuum bags
4. Look for wedding gift for cousin

Q: What is your ideal vacation?

1. Get the car washed
2. Renew your license
3. Pick up two gallons of milk
4. Get prices on blinds for family room

Q: What would you like to accomplish in the next year?

1. Renew magazine subscription
2. Buy software program for computer
3. Drop off VCR at repair shop
4. Purchase four blank videotapes

Q: Who in your life has had the biggest influence on you?

1. Buy printer ribbon for computer printer
2. Call in meter reading to gas company
3. Inquire about airfares to San Francisco and Paris
4. Buy a gift certificate for your sister's birthday

Q: Who is somebody famous that you admire? Why?

1. Call to reserve book at bookstore
2. Exchange blouse for a different color
3. Take pants to the tailor
4. Send flowers to friend in hospital

Q: How do you feel about charities? Which do you like most?

1. Call to have washing machine serviced
2. Change batteries in smoke detectors
3. Put advertisement in newspaper for child care
4. Order new checks

Q: How might you volunteer your time to help someone?

1. Check furnace filter and change, if needed
2. Call dealership to schedule service on your car brakes
3. Call dentist's office for evening appointment
4. Clean out fireplace

Q: What are four qualities an ideal friend would possess?

FUNCTIONAL MEMORY TASK
RECALL OF SITUATIONAL DETAILS

PURPOSE:

The purpose of this task is to improve the client's ability to recall detailed verbal information regarding functional situations.

DIRECTIONS:

The client is required to listen to verbally presented situational passages. Recall of specific information is assessed through use of questions.

TO INCREASE TASK DIFFICULTY:

1. Increase the number of passages presented for recall.

2. Increase length and complexity of passage information to recall (e.g., add details such as color, number of objects, specific locations).

PRIMARY SKILLS TARGETED:

1. Encoding of Information

2. Storage of Information

3. Retrieval of Information

4. Sustained Attention

TO ADDRESS THE RELATED SKILL OF:	**INCORPORATE THIS TASK MODIFICATION:**
1. Speed of Retrieval	Impose time constraint (e.g., recall passage information as quickly as possible)
2. Speed of Processing	Present information at a fast rate
3. Selective Attention	Complete task in a distracting environment (e.g., talk radio, others talking in background)
4. Delayed Recall	Have client answer an unrelated question or complete another task prior to recall of the information

PERFORMANCE MEASURES:

Evaluate the following:

■ Amount of passage information accurately recalled as indicated by percentage of recall questions answered accurately

■ Ability to recall passage information following another task

■ Need for repetition of paragraph in order to successfully encode

■ Effect of task modification(s) on performance (e.g., speed, distractions)

FUNCTIONAL PASSAGES FOR RECALL

1. Kathy had several errands to complete this past weekend. She needed to pick up clothing at the dry cleaners, return a library book, get a prescription filled, and cash her check. Unfortunately, the dry cleaners and bank were closed.

   What errands did she complete?

   What errands must she complete tomorrow?

2. Carol needs to drive her son's car pool today. She must pick up Jerry, Keith, Peter, and Daniel. Unknown to her, Peter was sick and would not be going to school.

   Who did she end up driving to school?

3. Mike needs to order two pizzas for his family—one for his two daughters and son and one for his wife and himself. He ordered a large pepperoni and cheese pizza for his wife and himself and a medium mushroom, pepperoni, and green pepper pizza for his kids.

   What items are on the large pizza?

   How many people are eating pizza?

   What items are on the medium pizza?

4. After going to the bank, Bryan and Laura reviewed the loan figures for refinancing their mortgage. For a 30-year mortgage, they could get a loan at 6½% with two points or 7% with no points. For a 15-year mortgage, they could get a loan at 6% with two points or 6½% with no points. They decided to go with the highest interest rate.

   How many years will their mortgage be?

   How many points will they have to pay?

5. Mina, a young mother, was going to make a healthy snack for her daughter's class at school. She needed to buy stick pretzels, small chocolate chips, granola, and peanut butter.

   What is the healthy snack for?

   What ingredients does she need to buy?

6. To transfer the title of his car into his name, Simon had to have an emissions' test done on his car. He also needed to bring a copy of his insurance policy to the Secretary of State's office with proof of the emissions' test.

   What two things did Simon need to bring into the Secretary of State?

   What was Simon attempting to do?

7. While planning a surprise baby shower for her friend, Regina had to decide on a guest list, buy invitations, send out the invitations, decide on a luncheon menu, and order a special cake. Fortunately, two friends were able to help plan the party.

   What things must be done for the party?

   Why is Regina giving the party?

   How many people will be helping Regina with the party?

8. On the way home from work, Alex stopped at the dry cleaners to pick up his dry cleaning, bought a salad from the deli, mailed a package at the post office, and tried to rent a movie but the one he wanted was not available.

   When did Alex do his errands?

   What errands did he do?

   What was Alex unable to do?

9. Before going to their friends' wedding, Ken and Koleen had to buy a card, wrap the gift, check the map for directions to the church, and put film in their camera. Even after checking the map, they got lost on the way to the church, making it to the ceremony just after the bride walked down the aisle.

   What did Ken and Koleen do to get ready for the wedding?

   What happened on the way to the church?

   When did they arrive at the ceremony?

10. Five friends planned to get together for the Super Bowl. Tami was going to bring the taco dip, Jim ordered a huge submarine sandwich, Robin baked cookies, Matt bought several kinds of soda pop, and Sara made a large tossed salad.

    How many friends got together?

    Why did they plan the gathering?

    What did the afternoon's menu consist of?

11. Last night, Monica did two loads of laundry, ironed her husband's shirts, sent e-mail to her best friend and a colleague, called her mom, and made a dessert for the next evening's card party. She had to leave a message on her mother's answering machine and made a note to herself to buy decorative napkins for the party.

    Whom did Monica talk to on the telephone?

    What does she need to buy for the party?

    What other activities did Monica complete last night?

    How did Monica remind herself to buy napkins?

12. While walking, Ben and Hillary saw three swans at the pond, six new houses being built, and a neighbor running with his dog. They stopped for frozen yogurt on the way home. Ben ordered pineapple and banana, while Hillary had a chocolate and vanilla swirl.

    What did Ben and Hillary see while walking?

    Why did they stop on the way home?

    Who ordered which yogurt flavors?

13. Sasha decided to take the train to Chicago to visit her brother and several friends. First, she called the train station to find out the cost of the ride and various departure and arrival times. Then she made arrangements for someone to take her to the train station and for someone to pick her up in Chicago. Lastly, Sasha packed an overnight bag and took off for the weekend.

    Who was Sasha going to visit?

    What did she do first to plan her trip?

    What city was she visiting?

14. Before buying a big screen T.V., Zach comparison shopped at three different stores, trying to find the best price. He finally decided on a 53" Sony television with a remote control.

    What size television did Zach want to buy?

    How many stores did he go to?

    What kind of television did he end up buying?

15. Jennifer needs to prepare to move by packing her belongings, calling the telephone company to shut off her telephone, and changing her address at the post office. She forgot to ask the movers to bring boxes and she did not call to have her electricity bill transferred to her new address.

    Who is this paragraph about?

    Which tasks did she need to complete?

    Which task took the least amount of time to get done?

    Which tasks did she forget to complete?

16. Angela is planning a surprise 30th birthday party for her husband Rick. The children are responsible for making the decorations. Angela will write out the invitations and prepare the food. She plans to invite 40 people and have the party on a weekend during the day.

    What type of party is Angela planning?

    What tasks does she need to complete?

    Who is she planning to have assist her with the preparations?

    When will she have the party?

17. Pauline is planning her annual vacation. In previous years, she went to California, Massachusetts, and Hawaii. This year, she wishes to go international, to France and Switzerland. In addition to her airplane ticket, she will need a passport and a train pass. She has already purchased a new backpack and a French pocket dictionary.

   Where has Pauline previously traveled?

   Where is she going this year?

   What has she already purchased?

   What does she still need to buy?

18. Janet needs to go to the library. She would like to find a book on gardening for herself, a book on photography for her husband, and a book on dogs for her daughters. She was only able to find books for herself and her daughters.

   Where was Janet going?

   What type of book did she want for herself?

   What are the topics of the books she found?

   What book was she unable to find?

19. While at the store, Lowell found two pairs of pants, returned a sweater, and exchanged a coat for a different size. He did not have enough cash, so he wrote a check for the difference. On the way home, he got a flat tire. Fortunately, he had road service through his insurer and was able to get assistance.

   What items did Lowell bring home?

   How did he pay for the items?

   What happened on the way home?

   How was the problem resolved?

20. Josh went in for his annual doctor's visit. The following week, he received his test results. The doctor reported that Josh had a normal EKG, but elevated cholesterol and blood pressure. He recommended medication, diet modification, and exercise to address these problems. Josh was asked to return to the doctor in 3 months.

   How long did it take for Josh to get his test results?

   What were the test results?

   What did the doctor recommend?

   When does Josh need to return to the doctor?

FUNCTIONAL MEMORY TASK

DELAYED RECALL

PURPOSE:

The purpose of this task is to improve the client's ability to recall requested items or learned information after a lengthy delay to promote effective compensatory strategy use.

DIRECTIONS:

Ask the client to either recall information learned or discussed during the previous therapy session or remember to bring in an item requested by the clinician. Initially, inform the client that, to enhance recall of specific information, he or she will be required to recall any information shared during the present therapy session in the next therapy session. The client is allowed to independently utilize any compensatory strategies to assist with recall (e.g., take notes, highlight information).

TO INCREASE TASK DIFFICULTY:

1. Increase the amount of information to be recalled (e.g., number of details).
2. Gradually increase the time delay (e.g., 1 day, 3 days, 1 week) prior to recall of the previous information.
3. Increase the number of topics and related information to be recalled.

PRIMARY SKILLS TARGETED:

1. Functional Memory (information storage and retrieval)
2. Prospective Memory
3. Sustained Attention
4. Functional Memory
5. Initiation and Self-Monitoring of Strategy Use

TO ADDRESS THE RELATED SKILL OF: INCORPORATE THIS TASK MODIFICATION:

1. Selective Attention

Have the client recall information in the presence of distractions (e.g., talk radio, others talking in background)

PERFORMANCE MEASURES:

Evaluate the following:

■ Ability to recall item(s) or information following a time delay

■ Percentage of information completely recalled after the delay

■ Percentage of information completely recalled with additional cues provided

■ Successful use of compensatory strategies

■ Effect of task modification(s) on performance (e.g., distractions)

ITEMS TO RECALL

Ask the client to bring a specific object from home to the next therapy session. (Ascertain that the client has such an object at home, so it is not necessary to buy the object.) To increase complexity, increase the number of objects to be recalled.

favorite book or magazine

family picture

stamped envelope

specific amount of change

personal item of choice

specific item of clothing

an object of a certain color

one left shoe

favorite recipe

special object

baseball hat

blank greeting card

one earring

necktie

colored sock

other objects of personal relevance to the client

INFORMATION TO RECALL

■ Recall information learned during the previous therapy session.

Examples:

topics of discussion

tasks completed

new facts

new word(s) learned

specific information from articles presented verbally or in writing

■ Recall information discussed by the client during the previous therapy session.

Examples:

a point of concern that was discussed

a positive event or personal accomplishment

a question or concern with work or school

a question or concern regarding therapy tasks

a personal goal

FUNCTIONAL MEMORY TASK

UNDERSTANDING YOUR MEMORY FUNCTIONING

PURPOSE:

The purpose of this task is to educate the client regarding his or her prospective memory functioning, and the importance of "remembering to remember." Improved prospective memory will better enable your client to complete a specific task at a designated time. This task will increase self-awareness of limitations in this often impaired skill area, which will promote successful use of individualized compensatory strategies.

DIRECTIONS:

Provide and review the definitions of each memory term as presented on the following pages. Have the client place a check next to each task that is difficult to recall and complete. Tally the total number of **p**'s (prospective memory examples) and the total number of **r**'s (retrospective memory examples). Further review the two different types of memory recall and related compensatory strategies to provide the client with ways to enhance these specific memory functions.

PRIMARY SKILLS TARGETED:

1. Prospective memory

2. Self-awareness

PERFORMANCE MEASURES:

Evaluate the following:

■ Average number of prospective memory examples checked

■ Average number of retrospective memory examples checked

PROSPECTIVE MEMORY TASKS

Definition

Remembering to carry out intended actions in the future at a specified time.

Examples

1. Remember to make a telephone call later in the day
2. Remember to complete a specific task tomorrow
3. Remember a doctor's appointment tomorrow

Remembering to complete a specific task in the future involves more planning, organization, and self-monitoring skills than recalling something that happened in the past. Prospective memory tasks also require more cognitive effort and attention in order to recall the details (what, when, where) of the specified task or action.

Source: Adapted from Fahy, J. F., and Schmitter, M. E. (1991). Current issues in memory research: What is prospective memory? *The Journal of Head Injury, 2*(4), 38–41.

RETROSPECTIVE MEMORY

Definition

Ability to remember past events

Examples

1. Recalling a musical concert you attended in the past

2. Remembering two activities you did last weekend

3. Recalling where you went to high school and what year you graduated

Remembering a past event or experience requires less cognitive effort than using your prospective memory (remembering to remember). Retrospective memory simply requires you to retrieve past events and experiences from long-term storage.

Source: Adapted from Fahy, J. F., and Schmitter, M. E. (1991). Current issues in memory research: What is prospective memory? *The Journal of Head Injury,* 2(4), 38–41.

MEMORY CHECKLIST

Name: _____

Date: _____

Directions:

Please place a check next to each item that is difficult for you to remember. Then tally the total number of p's checked and the total number of r's. Review these results with your clinician.

_____ Recalling an old favorite song (r)

_____ Turning off your headlights (p)

_____ Checking gas and oil gauge before a trip (p)

_____ Recognizing an old friend (r)

_____ Turning on the oven to bake (p)

_____ Remembering a person's name (r)

_____ Mailing a birthday card (p)

_____ Remembering a telephone number (r)

_____ Remembering your last vacation (r)

_____ Taking medication or vitamins after a meal (p)

_____ Setting an alarm clock for a specific time (p)

_____ Scheduling your next doctor appointment (p)

_____ Remembering a specific job instruction (r)

_____ Remembering where your high school graduation took place (r)

_____ Regularly attending a monthly meeting (p)

_____ Remembering to go to a dental appointment (p)

_____ Setting a stove timer (p)

_____ Recalling your favorite childhood book (r)

_____ Purchasing tickets for an upcoming event (p)

Source: Adapted from Fahy, J. F., and Schmitter, M. E. (1991). Current issues in memory research: What is prospective memory? *The Journal of Head Injury 2*(4), 38–41.

_____ Recognizing relatives in family pictures (r)

_____ Recalling your first job position (r)

TOTAL NUMBER OF P'S (PROSPECTIVE MEMORY EXAMPLES): _____

TOTAL NUMBER OF R'S (RETROSPECTIVE MEMORY EXAMPLES): _____

PROSPECTIVE MEMORY TASK
TASK COMPLETION WITH TIME CUES

PURPOSE:

The purpose of this task is to improve the client's ability to remember to complete activities in the future when provided time cues.

DIRECTIONS:

Present the client with one or two prospective memory tasks provided on the following page to complete throughout the therapy session. Instruct the client to use newly learned compensatory strategies to assist with completion of each task. Continue with other therapy activities, noting if client completes the requested task at the specified time.

TO INCREASE TASK DIFFICULTY:

1. Increase the number of tasks to complete throughout the therapy session.
2. Gradually increase the length of time between presentation and completion of the task.
3. Increase the complexity of the task to carry out at the specific time.

PRIMARY SKILLS TARGETED:

1. Prospective Memory
2. Retention of Information
3. Divided Attention
4. Self-monitoring of Strategy Use

PERFORMANCE MEASURES:

Evaluate the following:

- Percentage of presented tasks completed correctly at the requested time
- Percentage of presented tasks completed correctly with additional cues
- Successful use of compensatory memory strategies

TASKS WITH TIME CUES

"Work on this task for _____ minutes."

"Let me know when there are _____ minutes left in the therapy session."

"When your watch says _____, stop the task."

"When your watch says _____, ask me a question."

"When you have worked for _____ minutes, put down your pen."

"Meet me here [specific location known to the client] tomorrow."

"At the end of each month, send me a _____."

"During the middle of the session, tell me the time."

"Call me on [date] at [time]."

"Put your home tasks on my desk prior to our therapy session."

"Send me a note during your vacation.

"At [time] remind me to _____."

"Before you leave, ask [specific person] if you may use the phone to call home."

"Let me know when there is 5 minutes left in the therapy session."

"Find out one of the following and either tell me during our next therapy session or call me on [date] at [time]."

    1. weekend weather

    2. cost of a flight to a destination of interest

    3. price of a specified item

    4. location of a specific store

    5. the time and channel of a televised event of interest

    6. two facts from the news or newspaper

    7. date of an upcoming sporting event, concert, etc.

    8. cost of an upcoming play, concert, etc.

    9. store that stocks a book or computer program of personal interest

  10. other information of personal relevance to the client

PROSPECTIVE MEMORY TASK

TASK COMPLETION WITH ASSOCIATIVE CUES

PURPOSE:

The purpose of this task is to improve the client's ability to remember to complete activities in the future when provided associative cues.

DIRECTIONS:

Present the client with one or two prospective memory tasks provided on the following page to complete throughout the therapy session. Instruct the client to use newly learned compensatory strategies to assist with completion of each task. Continue with other therapy activities, noting if client completes the requested task when the associative cue is presented.

TO INCREASE TASK DIFFICULTY:

1. Increase the number of tasks to complete throughout the therapy session.
2. Gradually increase the length of time prior to presenting the associative cue for completion of the task.
3. Increase the complexity of the task to carry out when the associative cue is presented.
4. Increase the number of tasks to complete when the associative cue is presented.

PRIMARY SKILLS TARGETED:

1. Prospective Memory
2. Divided Attention
3. Retention of Information
4. Self-Monitoring of Strategy Use

TO ADDRESS THE RELATED SKILL OF: INCORPORATE THIS TASK MODIFICATION:

1. Alternating Attention   Alternate the response required when following the same associative cue

PERFORMANCE MEASURES:

Evaluate the following:

- Percentage of presented tasks completed correctly when the associative cue is presented
- Percentage of presented tasks completed correctly with additional cues
- Successful use of compensatory memory strategies
- Effect of task modification(s) on performance (e.g., speed, distractions, change in focus)

TASK WITH ASSOCIATIVE CUES

"Each time I show you this picture, take it and turn it over."

"Each time I open the door, hand me your pencil."

"When I stand up, write the date on this piece of paper."

"Whenever I ask you a question, say my name prior to answering."

"When you see me writing with a red pen, you switch to using a pencil."

"When I scratch my arm, repeat the task instructions."

"When you walk out of the therapy room, tell me one thing you need to complete this week."

"Each time I open this folder, place a sheet of paper in it."

"Each time I open this book, tell me something enjoyable you did this week."

"Each time I fold my hands, fold your hands."

"Whenever I drink some water, hand me the paper you are working on."

"When I cough once, ignore it. When I cough twice, cross your arms."

"Whenever I tap my pencil on the table, write your name."

"Whenever I sigh, write your zip code."

Instruct the client to listen for verbal use of a specific word or phrase throughout the therapy session. Word examples include: "strategies," "functional," "good job," "task," and so on. Upon hearing the word or phrase, the client is required to place a check mark or tally on a sheet of paper. Clinician and client should compare the total number at the end of the session.

HOME PRACTICE TASKS

Several of the ideas listed below can be completed during the monitoring period of treatment, with the clinician recording client performance. Other ideas can be suggested to the client on discharge for continued stimulation to promote maintenance of therapy gains.

- While watching news segments, generate two key words to assist with recall of information to discuss with family member or friend

- Video- or audiotape a segment of the news from radio or television and summarize in writing what you remember. Then, review the tape and compare information to check recall. After reading a section of a magazine article, newspaper, or book, summarize the key points to yourself or a family member

- At the end of the day, take 10 minutes to recall and discuss your activities and events of the day. Attempt to recall specific information such as the time you completed a particular activity, the location of the activity, the people you were with including unfamiliar people, problems you encountered, and any new information you learned

- Prepare for the next day by recalling tasks still needing completion, as well as other responsibilities to be completed tomorrow

- Recall your weekly list of to-do's and compare to written list for accuracy

- Recall current month's family and friends' birthdays and check your calendar for accuracy

- At the beginning of the week, recall and discuss three to five enjoyable or educational activities you completed the previous week

- At the end of the week, recall three to five people whom you talked to during the week; to increase difficulty, attempt to recall the topic of discussion

- Plan a date in the near future to send a letter or pay bills and attempt to remember to complete the tasks without any external cues

SUGGESTIONS FOR FAMILIES

■ Give your family member time to "remember" the word or item he or she is attempting to recall

■ Cue your family member to describe the word, idea, or event he or she is attempting to retrieve (e.g., "Use other words")

■ Be sure to include your family member when discussing and reminiscing about past events to assist with recall

■ Help your family member clarify his or her recalled thoughts by asking a variety of questions regarding the event or appointment

■ Allow your family member to explain information (even if it is not completely clear or organized) to give opportunities for practice and confidence-building.

■ Keep items such as car keys, umbrella, and calendar in designated places to provide organization for improved recall of location

■ Utilize electronic devices such as pagers, answering machines, and computers to leave messages and write lists for your family member

■ Ask about therapy, skill areas addressed, and improvements

■ Ask about successful compensatory strategies used by your family member

■ Encourage your family member to utilize compensatory memory strategies

■ Realize your family member may have difficulty with recall of daily events and recently learned information, despite long-term memory for preinjury events being fully intact

■ Be patient and sensitive

CHAPTER 6

Treating Word Retrieval and Thought Formulation Impairments

DEFINITIONS

Word Retrieval

A cognitive-language skill requiring the ability to effectively store and readily access words to clearly convey one's thoughts, feelings, and opinions. At the most basic level, this skill allows one to accurately name concrete concepts such as objects. At a higher level, this skill allows one to precisely describe more abstract concepts at a rapid rate.

Thought Formulation

A cognitive-language skill requiring the ability to readily access, retain, and organize words and concepts into verbal or written sentences to clearly convey one's thoughts and ideas, in order to fulfill a variety of communication purposes.

Specific to the mild-to-moderate TBI population, impairments in these skill areas may manifest themselves in difficulties such as:

- Inaccurate naming or non-specific descriptions
- Delayed access of desired words, particularly in the context of a conversation
- Decreased encoding, retention, and recall due to difficulty using cue words to store and access information
- Reduced organization and clarity of verbal or written comments and statements
- Ineffective verbal or written formulation and expression of higher level information

OTHER CONTRIBUTING COGNITIVE IMPAIRMENTS

Cognitive impairments that may be seen in people with mild-to-moderate TBI which may result in **word retrieval** difficulties:

Difficulties with:	May lead to:
1. Attention	Fluctuations in attention leading to a delay in word retrieval for thought formulation and expression
	Interruption of the search process for target word(s) due to fluctuating attention
2. Organization	Erratic word search pattern
	Reduced sequencing, categorization, and storage of word associations
3. Memory	Difficulty encoding and retaining specific information
	Difficulty accessing stored information
4. Cognitive Flexibility	Limited ability to consider alternative word choices to clearly express ideas
5. Divergent Thinking	Difficulty accessing various word choices in order to retrieve precise target word(s)

Cognitive impairments that may be seen in people with mild-to-moderate TBI which may result in **thought formulation** difficulties:

Difficulties with:	**May lead to:**
1. Attention	
a. sustained	Losing direction or train of thought
b. selective	Losing train of thought or experiencing difficulty with formulating one's thoughts due to the interference of internal or external distractions
c. alternating	Difficulty in switching between ideas or topics during ongoing dialogue
d. divided	Difficulty engaging in conversation while completing other basic tasks
2. Speed of Processing	Reduced rate of accessing specific words and formulating thoughts and opinions, while alternately listening or responding to others' conversational comments
3. Organization	Difficulty sequencing words into meaningful sentences and logically organizing thoughts for expression
4. Working Memory	Difficulty retaining selected words and thoughts long enough to express oneself verbally or in writing
5. Word Retrieval	Limitations in accessing specific words necessary to clearly and concisely express connected thoughts and ideas
6. Elaboration	Reduced ability to expand one's thoughts, comments, and opinions for a more comprehensive explanation
7. Cognitive Flexibility	Limited ability to maintain a broad range of thoughts in order to consider multiple viewpoints and expression options and to readily select alternative statements to convey ideas or opinions
8. Divergent Thinking	Difficulty generating various and multiple ideas for meaningful discourse

FUNCTIONAL IMPLICATIONS OF WORD RETRIEVAL AND THOUGHT FORMULATION IMPAIRMENTS

The following is a list of many of the abilities needed for successful communication in the natural environments of home, work, and school. Impairments in word retrieval and thought formulation in people with mild-to-moderate TBI may present communication concerns that compromise performance in these functional environments. You are encouraged to explore these and other related activities with your clients to create functional and personally relevant therapy tasks and to maximize carryover of therapeutic gains to the natural environment.

In the Home

Ability to...

■ **Effectively communicate one's feelings and opinions**

Examples:

Resolve family conflicts

Respond to questions from spouse, children, and other family members

Discuss important issues related to personal or family goals

Discuss current events and daily issues

Resolve issues with neighbors

■ **Effectively communicate factual information**

Examples:

Discuss television or radio news reports

Discuss newspaper and magazine articles

Explain information regarding home repairs

Relay doctor's recommendations or other medical advice

Communicate telephone messages to others

■ **Effectively communicate on the telephone**

Examples:

Discuss complaints and concerns

Resolve utility or financial bill problems

Ask consumer questions or request information

Engage in social conversation

Schedule appointments and meetings

Discuss prescription information with pharmacist

At Work

Ability to...

■ **Effectively communicate to clearly express oneself for job task completion and vocational success**

Examples:

Explain complex information

Request specific information

Ask or answer questions verbally or in writing

Participate in discussion (for work-related and social purposes)

Express opinions and ideas

Relay relevant thoughts and comments

Draft company memos

Prepare and verbally present information (speeches)

Facilitate meetings

Voice concerns and complaints

Mediate complaints or problems

Train others or provide instruction

Write or verbally present reports

Discuss information over the telephone

Report facts and figures

At School

Ability to...

■ **Effectively communicate for social interaction (consider issues of embarrassment, frustration, and isolation)**

Examples:

Form peer relationships

Develop study sessions with others

Interact with teachers or professors

Participate in group projects

Participate in student social activities

Request assistance or explanations

■ **Effectively communicate verbally and in writing for academic success**

Examples:

Take notes

Complete homework assignments

Complete essay tests

Write papers

Give impromptu speeches

Take oral exams

Ask and respond to questions

Explain homework

Provide facts and opinions

Participate in classroom discussion

In addition to the word-retrieval tasks provided in the following pages, you may utilize the information listed above to create unique therapy tasks that will be most meaningful for your client, depending on his or her goal environment. Please refer to the cover sheet for each task to assist you with addressing related skills simultaneously.

COMPENSATORY STRATEGIES

Select from this list the word-retrieval and thought formulation strategies that would be most helpful for and effectively utilized by your clients, considering their skill limitations and potential home, work, and school environments. It is recommended that these strategies be taught to the client and incorporated into the therapy sessions until the client is able to utilize them successfully and independently. Additionally, allow for practice of the specific strategy in the target environment to ensure successful carryover.

The following strategies may assist clients in retrieving desired words and assist listeners in understanding the intended meaning:

- Attempt to describe the word (i.e., appearance, location, function)

- Attempt to make an association with something familiar

- Utilize gestures and nonverbal communication

- Consider various associated categories or subcategories of the intended word

- Attempt to retrieve a synonym or antonym for the word

- Visualize a picture or spelling of the word

- Visualize a relevant scene or event to increase thought generation

- Imagine someone else saying the word in a previous conversation

- Indicate the need for a momentary pause to allow time to access the word or thought

- Use a time delay and self-talk to relax yourself for enhanced word retrieval or thought access

- Attempt to generate a carrier phrase to stimulate word recall or thought completion

- When learning a new name, attempt to utilize or repeat the name in conversation several times

- When learning a new name, attempt to associate the name with a well-known personality or someone familiar to you

- Do not avoid a word you are not able to readily retrieve, as this may impact your ability to recall the word in the future

- If, after using any or all of these strategies, you are still unable to recall a specific word or thought, attempt to recall it later when you are in a different setting and more relaxed

WORD-RETRIEVAL TASK
CATEGORY NAMING

PURPOSE:

The purpose of this task is to improve the client's ability to rapidly access and name items in uncommon categories.

DIRECTIONS:

Present the client with a specific category and instruct him or her to name multiple members of the category as quickly as possible, beginning with three members per category and increasing up to ten. Categories may be presented on index cards as a visual reminder.

TO INCREASE THE DIFFICULTY:

1. Disallow certain obvious responses (e.g., for the category "something that is grown," do not allow names of foods).

2. Disallow members from the same subcategory; require more diversity (e.g., allow the name of *one* beverage for "something that is spilled" rather than several).

3. Request members that would fit in two categories (e.g., name "something that is blue and can be spilled").

PRIMARY SKILLS TARGETED:

1. Rapid Word Retrieval

2. Divergent Thinking

3. Sustained Attention

TO ADDRESS THE RELATED SKILL OF:	INCORPORATE THIS TASK MODIFICATION:
1. Speed of Retrieval	Impose time constraint (e.g., client to provide as many items as possible in a set amount of time)
2. Selective Attention	Complete task in a distracting environment (e.g., news talk radio, others talking in background, seated near window)
3. Alternating Attention	Select two categories and require client to alternately name a member from each category (e.g., something that is painted, something that is loud, something that is painted, something that is loud ...)

PERFORMANCE MEASURES:

Evaluate the following:

- Average number of words or ideas generated in predetermined time frame
- Maximum number of words or ideas generated in predetermined time frame
- Ability to provide creative responses
- Ability to provide diverse responses
- Effect of task modification(s) on performance (e.g., speed, distractions, change in focus)

NAME THINGS THAT ARE . . .

1. cut

2. warm

3. salty

4. torn

5. scary

6. folded

7. washed

8. breakable

9. loud

10. pulled

11. pushed

12. poured

13. held in your hand

14. hard to spell

15. easy to lose

16. plugged in

17. brushed

18. wet

19. plastic

20. dangerous

21. opened

22. discarded

23. difficult to do

24. tiny

25. growing

26. blue

27. listened to

28. smooth

29. spilled

30. stirred

31. locked up

32. walked on

33. climbed

34. worn

35. cooked

36. painted

37. driven

38. developed

39. disappointing

40. pleasing

41. built

42. relaxing

43. evaluated

44. produced

45. taught

46. controversial

47. reviewed

48. compressed

49. fun

50. closed

51. expensive

52. saved for

53. painful

54. sad

55. rejuvenating

56. borrowed

57. sweet

58. prepared

59. censored

60. edited

WORD-RETRIEVAL TASK
GENERATING SYNONYMS

PURPOSE:

The purpose of this task is to improve the client's ability to access diverse, synonymous higher level words.

DIRECTIONS:

1. Present the client with four target words, one at a time, and ask the client to verbally generate as many synonyms as possible for each.

2. Then provide the client with the same target words to brainstorm in writing at home.

3. Retest on the same target words verbally 1 week later.

PRIMARY SKILLS TARGETED:

1. Higher Level Word Retrieval

2. Divergent Thinking

3. Accessing Words Through Verbal and Written Modalities

TO ADDRESS THE RELATED SKILL OF: INCORPORATE THIS TASK MODIFICATION:

1. Speed of Processing — Impose time constraint during verbal portion

2. Selective Attention — Complete task in a distracting environment (e.g., news talk radio, others talking in background, visually stimulating environment)

3. Alternating Attention — After retesting, provide target words in an alternating fashion, having the client quickly generate a synonym for each (e.g., Target #1, #2, #3, #1, #4)

PERFORMANCE MEASURES:

Evaluate the following:

■ Number of words generated in each modality (compare)

■ Number of words generated after multi-modality stimulation

■ Effect of task modification(s) on performance (e.g., distractions, speed)

■ Impact of stress and time issues when performing at home versus during the therapy session

GENERATING SYNONYMS

Directions: Try to generate as many synonyms as you can.

1. loud

First trial: _____

_____

_____

_____

One week later: _____

_____

_____

_____

2. original

First trial: _____

_____

_____

_____

One week later _____

_____

_____

_____

3. ornate

First trial: _____

_____

GENERATING SYNONYMS

_____

_____

One week later: _____

_____

_____

_____

4. courageous

First trial: _____

_____

_____

One week later: _____

_____

_____

_____

5. combine

First trial: _____

_____

_____

_____

GENERATING SYNONYMS

One week later: _____

_____

_____

_____

6. energetic

First trial: _____

_____

_____

_____

One week later: _____

_____

_____

_____

7. authorize

First trial: _____

_____

_____

_____

One week later: _____

_____

GENERATING SYNONYMS

_____

_____

8. anxious

First trial: _____

_____

_____

_____

One week later: _____

_____

_____

_____

9. injured

First trial: _____

_____

_____

One week later: _____

_____

_____

GENERATING SYNONYMS

10. produce (verb)

First trial: _____

_____

_____

_____

One week later: _____

_____

_____

_____

11. patient (adjective)

First trial: _____

_____

_____

_____

One week later: _____

_____

_____

_____

12. nonchalant

First trial: _____

_____

GENERATING SYNONYMS

_____

_____

One week later: _____

_____

_____

_____

13. mature

First trial: _____

_____

_____

One week later: _____

_____

_____

14. magnify

First trial:_____

_____

_____

_____

GENERATING SYNONYMS

One week later: _____

_____

_____

_____

15. instill

First trial: _____

_____

_____

_____

One week later: _____

_____

_____

_____

16. intelligent

First trial: _____

_____

_____

_____

One week later: _____

_____

GENERATING SYNONYMS

_____

_____

17. necessary

First trial: _____

_____

_____

_____

One week later: _____

_____

_____

_____

18. eligible

First trial: _____

_____

_____

_____

One week later: _____

_____

_____

_____

GENERATING SYNONYMS

19. embarrassed

First trial: _____

_____

_____

_____

One week later: _____

_____

_____

_____

20. perfect

First trial: _____

_____

_____

_____

One week later: _____

_____

_____

_____

21. ridicule

First trial: _____

_____

GENERATING SYNONYMS

_____

_____

One week later: _____

_____

_____

_____

22. sensitive

First trial: _____

_____

_____

_____

One week later: _____

_____

_____

_____

23. personal

First trial: _____

_____

_____

_____

GENERATING SYNONYMS

One week later: _____

_____

_____

_____

24. obscure

First trial: _____

_____

_____

_____

One week later: _____

_____

_____

_____

25. hostile

First trial: _____

_____

_____

_____

One week later: _____

_____

GENERATING SYNONYMS

_____

_____

26. journey

First trial: _____

_____

_____

_____

One week later: _____

_____

_____

_____

27. clarify

First trial: _____

_____

_____

_____

One week later: _____

_____

_____

_____

GENERATING SYNONYMS

28. calculate

First trial: _____

_____

_____

_____

One week later: _____

_____

_____

_____

29. frivolous

First trial: _____

_____

_____

_____

One week later: _____

_____

_____

_____

30. finish

First trial: _____

_____

GENERATING SYNONYMS

_____

_____

One week later: _____

_____

_____

_____

HOME ASSIGNMENT

Write as many synonyms as you can. Please do not consult a thesaurus or dictionary.

1. loud

_____

_____

_____

_____

2. original

_____

_____

_____

_____

3. ornate

_____

_____

_____

_____

4. courageous

_____

_____

_____

_____

HOME ASSIGNMENT

Write as many synonyms as you can. Please do not consult a thesaurus or dictionary.

5. combine

_____

_____

_____

_____

6. energetic

_____

_____

_____

_____

7. authorize

_____

_____

_____

_____

8. anxious

_____

_____

_____

_____

HOME ASSIGNMENT

Write as many synonyms as you can. Please do not consult a thesaurus or dictionary.

9. injured

_____

_____

_____

_____

10. produce (verb)

_____

_____

_____

_____

11. patient (adjective)

_____

_____

_____

_____

12. nonchalant

_____

_____

_____

_____

HOME ASSIGNMENT

Write as many synonyms as you can. Please do not consult a thesaurus or dictionary.

13. mature

_____

_____

_____

_____

14. magnify

_____

_____

_____

_____

15. instill

_____

_____

_____

_____

16. intelligent

_____

_____

_____

_____

HOME ASSIGNMENT

Write as many synonyms as you can. Please do not consult a thesaurus or dictionary.

17. necessary

_____

_____

_____

_____

18. eligible

_____

_____

_____

_____

19. embarrassed

_____

_____

_____

_____

20. perfect

_____

_____

_____

_____

HOME ASSIGNMENT

Write as many synonyms as you can. Please do not consult a thesaurus or dictionary.

21. ridicule

_____

_____

_____

_____

22. sensitive

_____

_____

_____

_____

23. personal

_____

_____

_____

_____

24. obscure

_____

_____

_____

_____

HOME ASSIGNMENT

Write as many synonyms as you can. Please do not consult a thesaurus or dictionary.

25. hostile

_____

_____

_____

_____

26. journey

_____

_____

_____

_____

27. clarify

_____

_____

_____

_____

28. calculate

_____

_____

_____

_____

HOME ASSIGNMENT

Write as many synonyms as you can. Please do not consult a thesaurus or dictionary.

29. frivolous

_____

_____

_____

_____

30. finish

_____

_____

_____

_____

WORD-RETRIEVAL TASK

WORD ASSOCIATION

PURPOSE:

The purpose of this task is to improve the client's ability to access related higher level words.

DIRECTIONS:

Present the client with a target word, either verbally or on index cards, and instruct the client to either brainstorm as many words associated with the target word as quickly as possible (e.g., for *create* the client may say: build, make, painting, construct), or rapidly freely associate from one response to the next (e.g., for *create* the client may say: paint, artist, brush, hair).

TO INCREASE TASK DIFFICULTY:

1. Disallow common associations (e.g., for *celebration* do not allow *party*).

PRIMARY SKILLS TARGETED:

1. Higher Level Word Retrieval
2. Divergent Thinking

TO ADDRESS THE RELATED SKILL OF:	INCORPORATE THIS TASK MODIFICATION:
1. Speed of Processing	Impose time constraint, gradually reducing time allowed
2. Selective Attention	Complete task in a distracting environment (e.g., news talk radio, others talking in background, visual distractions)
3. Alternating Attention	Alternate brainstorming between two target words, presenting target words on index cards within the client's constant view (e.g., present the word *celebration*, then *organize*, then *celebration* again, then *organize* again, and so on)
4. Thought Elaboration	Have client explain various associations made (i.e., "Why did you associate *disappointment* with *celebration*?")

PERFORMANCE MEASURES:

Evaluate the following:

■ Number of words associated in predetermined time frame

■ Ability to be creative and extend thoughts beyond common associations (reasoning skills are required to make uncommon word associations)

■ Effect of task modification(s) on performance (e.g., impact of stress and time issues when associating words with distractions or under time constraints)

WORD ASSOCIATION

1. celebration
2. organize
3. explosion
4. motivated
5. mystery
6. embrace
7. fortunate
8. journey
9. frozen
10. fearful
11. nature
12. polluted
13. opportunity
14. process
15. deception
16. joyous
17. denial
18. jagged
19. theater
20. threatened
21. excited
22. expensive
23. career
24. smooth
25. approval
26. crowded

27. overwhelmed
28. reject
29. adventure
30. interview
31. humorous
32. doubtful
33. debate
34. trendy
35. impolite
36. disappearance
37. frustrated
38. struggle
39. create
40. wedding
41. music
42. budget
43. community
44. bankruptcy
45. calculate
46. challenge
47. anxiety
48. symphony
49. athlete
50. negative
51. criticize
52. environment

53. desolate

54. education

55. construction

56. sunshine

57. restaurant

58. mediate

59. imagine

60. appreciative

61. aging

62. addiction

63. hopeful

64. graduation

65. sympathy

66. medicine

67. peaceful

68. embarrass

69. chaos

70. dangerous

71. panic

72. wealthy

73. blizzard

74. encouragement

75. research

76. colleague

THOUGHT FORMULATION TASK
SENTENCE FORMULATION

PURPOSE:

The purpose of this task is to improve the client's ability to formulate thoughts in cohesive, complete sentences for improved verbal and written discourse.

DIRECTIONS:

Present the client with two words, either verbally or on index cards, gradually increasing the number of words, and instruct the client to formulate a sentence of at least eight words in length containing the target words.

TO INCREASE TASK DIFFICULTY:

1. Utilize more abstract stimulus words (e.g., adjectives).
2. Require a word minimum, gradually increasing the amount to lengthen the response, thus making it more descriptive.

PRIMARY SKILLS TARGETED:

1. Word Retrieval
2. Divergent Thinking
3. Thought Formulation
4. Sequencing and Organization

TO ADDRESS THE RELATED SKILL OF:	INCORPORATE THIS TASK MODIFICATION:
1. Speed of Processing	Limit formulation time allowed (e.g., 30 seconds to generate a sentence)
2. Selective Attention	Complete task in a distracting environment (e.g., others talking in background)
3. Cognitive Flexibility	Formulate a sentence with words in presented order, then switch order and have client formulate a new sentence with different meaning (e.g., 1. elevator, piano keys, laugh; 2. piano keys, laugh, elevator; 3. laugh, elevator, piano keys)
4. Thought Elaboration	Require client to generate more complex sentences of greater than 15 words

PERFORMANCE MEASURES:

Evaluate the following:

- Number of words generated per sentence

- Semantic correctness of the sentences

- Syntactic correctness of the sentences

- Effect of task modification(s) on performance (e.g., impact of stress and time issues when formulating thoughts with distractions or under time constraints)

SENTENCE FORMULATION

1. Select any combination of two words from the lists below.

2. To increase task complexity, select words that are not commonly associated.

elevator	calendar
piano keys	cherry pie
laugh	antenna
encyclopedia	camera
helicopter	pipe
scissors	verdict
jeans	organization
temperature	time
comb	sun
tractor	eagle
screwdriver	sweater
shoes	fire
bread	tornado
train	igloo
toast	business
late	trailer
kitchen	farm
reading	basketball
ambulance	blanket
shovel	marble
lightning	jury
frying pan	puzzle
pencil	coat
syrup	fish
raincoat	clock
airplane	rake
sink	river
bandaid	hairspray
frosting	dice
meeting	zipper
broom	key
promise	boots

SENTENCE FORMULATION

1. Select any combination of three words from the lists below.
2. To increase task complexity, select words that are not commonly associated.

eyelash	microscope	roof
spelling	glasses	thermometer
cuff	umbrella	mirror
corn	tricycle	soap
management	spatula	maple tree
future	fork	files
plant	television	wastebasket
grass	ticket	robe
whistle	stop sign	fingerprints
pillow	appetite	pretzel
mountains	map	hanger
envelope	flashlight	safety pin
haircut	flowers	telephone
restaurant	bird	vacation
stereo	skis	hawk
independence	oxygen	freedom
gold	jingle	toothbrush
error	chef	baggage
snow	beverage	computer
rain	listen	dinner
balance	violin	highway
president	association	brain
bridge	musical	marathon
strawberries	attic	stove
pressure	basement	towel
flu	fear	dessert
mall	driver	branch
warning	bagel	owner
desk	penguin	tourist
presentation	question	controversy
concern	baseball	announcement
union	taxi	jail
debate	editorial	autumn

THOUGHT FORMULATION TASK
THOUGHT GENERATION

PURPOSE:

The purpose of this task is to improve the client's ability to generate diverse ideas related by category and elaborate on these ideas, using detailed descriptions for improved thought retrieval, formulation, and expression.

DIRECTIONS:

Present the client with a specific action and instruct him or her to provide multiple, detailed descriptions of situations in which one might perform that action. Encourage creative and diverse responses. Begin by requiring three ideas per action and increase up to ten. Categories may be presented on index cards as a visual reminder.

TO INCREASE TASK DIFFICULTY:

1. Require a word minimum, gradually increasing the number to lengthen the response, thus making it more descriptive.

PRIMARY SKILLS TARGETED:

1. Organized Thought Formulation and Elaboration
2. Divergent Thinking
3. Sustained Attention

TO ADDRESS THE RELATED SKILL OF:	INCORPORATE THIS TASK MODIFICATION:
1. Speed of Retrieval	Impose time constraint for accessing each idea or several ideas as rapidly as possible (e.g., within 10 seconds)
2. Selective Attention	Complete task in a distracting environment (e.g., news talk radio, others talking in background, visually stimulating room)
3. Alternating Attention	Select two categories and require client to alternately name a situation for each category (e.g., a time when a person would jump, a time when a person would visit, a time when a person would jump, a time when a person would visit, and so on)

PERFORMANCE MEASURES:

Evaluate the following:

- Average number of ideas generated
- Maximum number of ideas generated
- Average length of response
- Maximum length of response
- Ability to provide creative responses
- Ability to provide detailed responses
- Ability to provide diverse responses
- Effect of task modification(s) on performance (e.g., speed, distractions, change in focus)

DESCRIBE SITUATIONS OR CONDITIONS WHEN ONE MIGHT:

1. celebrate

2. sweat

3. worry

4. lie

5. blink

6. scratch

7. scream

8. apologize

9. clean

10. protest

11. shop

12. sneeze

13. disagree

14. dance

15. yawn

16. beg

17. clap

18. yell

19. jump

20. bleed

21. laugh

22. cry

23. practice

24. run

25. hop

26. boo

27. sigh

28. complain

29. eat

30. call

31. shiver

32. visit

33. snoop

34. panic

35. give up

36. mourn

37. disappoint

38. agonize

39. threaten

40. scold

THOUGHT FORMULATION TASK
TOPIC DISCUSSION

PURPOSE:

The purpose of this task is to improve the client's ability to access, retain, and organize words and concepts into sentences to clearly convey thoughts for improved verbal and written discourse.

DIRECTIONS:

1. Present the client with a topic and ask the client to utilize the provided questions and ideas to stimulate an integrated, lengthy response.
2. Provide the client with the following page for reference to assist in developing a response.

PRIMARY SKILLS TARGETED:

1. Higher Level Word Retrieval
2. Divergent Thinking
3. Cognitive Flexibility
4. Thought Organization
5. Thought Formulation
6. Thought Elaboration

TO ADDRESS THE RELATED SKILL OF: INCORPORATE THIS TASK MODIFICATION:

1. Selective Attention — Complete task in a distracting environment (e.g., news talk radio, others talking in background, visual distractions)

2. Written Thought Formulation — Have the client provide a written response

PERFORMANCE MEASURES:

Evaluate the following:

- Ability to express thoughts in an organized, cohesive manner
- Ability to express thoughts clearly
- Ability to readily access desired words
- Ability to reason and think flexibly to understand multiple viewpoints
- Ability to think divergently to generate numerous ideas
- Effect of distractions on performance
- Responses in the verbal modality as compared to the written modality

QUESTIONS AND IDEAS TO GUIDE TOPIC DISCUSSION

Review these questions to assist you in formulating and responding, rather than directly answering each question.

1. When discussing both sides of the issue, include an explanation of why you think this topic is often a source of debate and division among people (i.e., What factors contribute to a person's viewpoint?). Consider the following factors:
   a. emotional
   b. intellectual
   c. cultural
   d. personal bias
   e. individual experiences

2. What may make a person take a stronger position?

3. What may make a person change his or her position?

4. Following an outline and discussion of both sides of the issue, summarize your viewpoint.

TOPICS FOR DISCUSSION

1. Political positions
2. Participating in war
3. A defendant's verdict
4. Television content
5. Raising children
6. Religious education
7. Racism and preferential treatment
8. Capital punishment
9. Media coverage
10. Abortion
11. Unions
12. Professional sports salaries
13. Welfare assistance
14. Defense spending
15. Foreign aid
16. Buying foreign imports
17. Government spending of tax dollars
18. Assisted suicide
19. Prayer in the public schools
20. Incarceration versus rehabilitation of criminals
21. Surrogacy
22. Rights of birth parents versus adoptive parents
23. Speed limits
24. Reporting crime by a family member
25. A "tough love" approach to parenting
26. Prolonging life through artificial means
27. Pornography
28. Working mothers
29. Women in the Armed Forces
30. Public employees with AIDS/HIV positive
31. Policing the Internet
32. Dating coworkers
33. Tabloid regulation
34. Personal opinions by news reporters
35. Homeopathic remedies

36. Vegetarianism
37. Gun control
38. Flag burning
39. Public service announcements promoting safe sex among teenagers
40. Classroom teaching via computer versus personal instruction by teacher
41. Mandatory bicycle and motorcycle helmets
42. Punishment for drunk drivers
43. Disciplining children
44. Legalizing marijuana
45. Social security system
46. Music censorship
47. Flat tax
48. Education in the public schools
49. Teenage pregnancy
50. Organic foods

HOME PRACTICE TASKS

Several of the ideas listed below can be completed during the monitoring period of treatment, with the therapist recording client performance. Other ideas may be suggested to the client on discharge to promote maintenance of therapy gains.

- At least once a day, engage in discussions of current events and other topics of interest

- Call family and friends on a regular basis

- Write letters to family and friends

- Volunteer as a facilitator of a group (e.g., parenting group, children's group, recipe club, support group, book review club)

- Take a speech class (or other adult education class)

- Keep a journal to record your thoughts and ideas

- Play word games such as Scrabble, Taboo, Boggle, Password

- Participate at home in televised game shows such as Jeopardy and Wheel of Fortune

- Watch a brief televised sitcom of interest and summarize a humorous incident for a family member or friend

- Complete crossword puzzles and word scrambles

- Write to the editor of a local newspaper or favorite magazine, expressing your opinion

- Read and discuss articles and books of interest with a friend or family member

- Handle daily responsibilities requiring telephone use to make inquiries or settle disputes

- If available, utilize a computer for word processing, vocabulary stimulation, and Internet communication

SUGGESTIONS FOR FAMILIES

■ Give your family member time to "find" the word for which he or she is searching

■ Do not provide the word for your family member unless asked or if you observe obvious frustration

■ Cue your family member to describe the word or idea he or she is trying to retrieve; for example, say, "use other words"

■ Be sure to include your family member in discussions; ask his or her suggestions, opinions, and ideas

■ Help your family member clarify his or her thoughts by asking a variety of questions

■ Allow your family member to explain information (even if it is not completely clear or organized) to provide opportunities for practice and confidence-building

■ Be patient and sensitive

■ Allow your family member to complete daily communication tasks such as returning telephone calls and scheduling appointments

■ Encourage your family member to utilize compensatory strategies learned in therapy

■ Allow your family member to request information while out in the community (e.g., stores, library, restaurant)

CHAPTER 7

Treating Information Processing Impairments (Auditory and Visual)

DEFINITION

Information Processing

A cognitive-language skill that relies on the abilities of perception, attention, comprehension, integration, retention, recall, and application of information presented in either the verbal or written modality (i.e., listening or viewing or reading). An impairment at any of these levels may interfere with the ability to accurately and efficiently process information necessary for learning purposes and daily functioning. More specifically, Kay and Silver (1988) state: "Head-injured persons often react more slowly, handle smaller amounts of information at one time, and take longer when required to cognitively process the information" (p. 69).

Specific to the mild-to-moderate TBI population, impairments in this skill area may manifest themselves in difficulties such as:

- Slowed speed of processing

- Reduced ability to process lengthy information accurately

- Limited ability to process complex information accurately

- Difficulty with sustaining attention, necessary for processing information

- Difficulty with selective attention, which may interfere with processing information in the presence of distractions

- Reduced working memory capacity, which may impact information retention, integration, and analysis

- Compromised ability to complete tasks due to reduced processing and decreased understanding of task directions

OTHER CONTRIBUTING COGNITIVE IMPAIRMENTS

Cognitive impairments seen in people with mild-to-moderate TBI that may result in **information processing** difficulties:

Difficulties with:	May lead to:
1. Attention	
a. sustained	Sensory overload, which interferes with accurate comprehension and retention of all presented information
b. alternating	Difficulty alternately attending to multiple ideas for integrated processing of information
	Difficulty switching attentional focus between processing information and executing another task
c. selective	Difficulty processing information due to interference from internal or external distractions

d. divided	Difficulty processing information while engaged in another task
2. Organization	Difficulty organizing incoming information which may result in reduced comprehension, retention, integration, and recall
3. Working Memory	Difficulty retaining information long enough to comprehend, integrate, and utilize facts and concepts
4. Speed of Processing	Delayed speed of processing, which may result in inaccurate perception, encoding, reception, and comprehension of information
5. Higher Level Reasoning	Difficulty comprehending and integrating complex, lengthy, and abstract information
6. Word Retrieval and Thought Formulation	Difficulty summarizing learned information verbally or in writing to assist with comprehension, retention, and application

FUNCTIONAL IMPLICATIONS OF INFORMATION PROCESSING IMPAIRMENTS

(Auditory and Visual)

The following is a list of many of the abilities needed for successful information processing in the natural environments of home, work, and school. Impairments in verbal and written information processing in people with mild-to-moderate TBI may compromise performance in these functional environments. You are encouraged to explore these and other related activities with your clients to create functional and personally relevant therapy tasks and to maximize carryover of therapeutic gains to the natural environment.

In the Home

Ability to...

■ **Effectively process information over the telephone**

Examples:

Discuss complaints and concerns

Resolve utility or financial bill problems

Ask consumer questions and obtain information

Engage in social conversation

Schedule appointments or arrange meetings

Obtain educational information

Obtain and record messages for self and others

■ **Effectively process factual information**

Examples:

Listen and discuss television and radio news reports

Obtain and relay doctor's recommendations and pertinent medical information

Review mail and determine requested action

Read and comprehend written material necessary for independent living

■ **Effectively process instructional information**

Examples:

Process verbal instructions for home repairs

Follow verbal directions to reach destinations

Read and follow written directions necessary for independent living

Review and process financial matters to provide needed information

■ **Effectively process others' feelings and opinions**

Examples:

Resolve family conflicts

Respond to questions from spouse, children, and other family members

Discuss important concerns related to personal or family issues

Discuss current events and daily issues

Discuss daily caregiver comments and concerns

Answer community questionnaires

Comprehend political issues

At Work

Ability to...

■ **Effectively process factual information for improved communication and follow up action**

Examples:

Understand messages from others

Process messages to relay to others

Read and follow written assignments

Review and discuss company memos and reports

Process specific questions and develop an appropriate response

Participate in ongoing discussions (work-related conversation, business or staff meetings, group projects)

■ **Effectively process instructional information for accurate task completion**

Examples:

Understand requests or instructions received from supervisor

Process and understand decisions and directions discussed at meetings

Read and follow instructional manuals for equipment

Read and comprehend professional resource material

Follow steps to successfully complete complex tasks

At School

Ability to...

■ **Accurately and efficiently process information for learning purposes**

Examples:

Take accurate class and lecture notes and integrate information

Review course texts and outline information

Discuss course information in study groups to improve new learning

Participate in group projects to fulfill course requirements

Participate in class discussions (ask and respond to questions)

Comprehend and complete course exams in a timely manner

In addition to the information processing tasks provided in the following pages, you may utilize the information listed above to create unique therapy tasks that will be most meaningful for your client, depending on his or her goals. Please refer to the cover sheet for each task to assist you with addressing related skills simultaneously.

COMPENSATORY STRATEGIES

Select from this list the information processing strategies that would be most useful for and effectively utilized by your clients, considering their skill limitations and potential home, work, and school environments. It is recommended that these strategies be taught to the client and incorporated into the therapy sessions until the client is able to utilize them successfully and independently. Additionally, allow for practice of the specific strategy in the target environment to ensure successful carryover.

Auditory (Encoding Verbal Information)

■ Eliminate auditory distractions in an effort to focus attention and enhance concentration while listening

■ Ask the speaker to slow down or to provide information in a shortened format

■ Request repetitions as needed and ask questions to confirm information or to clarify understanding

■ Utilize written notes to aid accuracy of information processing and retention

■ Paraphrase in your own words information heard

■ Use a tape recorder to record messages and important information

■ Write notes in an organized manner in an easily accessible datebook or notebook for consistent reference

■ Utilize self-questions to enhance understanding ("Did I understand what I heard?" "Does it make sense to me?" "Do I need the information repeated?")

■ Attempt to relate new information to personal experience or something already known

Visual (Decoding Visual Information)

■ Eliminate visual distractions in an effort to focus attention and enhance concentration while reading

■ Request additional time for reading and making organized notes

■ Use finger or index card to assist with maintaining place while scanning and reading information

■ Use a print blocker (index card, sheet of paper, etc.) to cover parts of the page, in order to focus on one section at a time

■ Write brief notes from reading material in your own words and organize topics for easy reference

■ Request explanations from others who may have a thorough knowledge of the topic you are reading

■ Verbalize or write summary statements after reading paragraphs or sections of the material

■ After a break, review notes before resuming reading to enhance integration of material read previously

INFORMATION PROCESSING TASK
INFORMATION PROCESSING SURVEY:
IMPORTANCE OF INFORMATION TO YOU

There are many different kinds of information to process: factual, explanatory, persuasive, sequential, argumentative, instructional, and leisure. Thus, it is important to know what types of information are most important to you and relevant to your activities of daily living or work responsibilities. Please take a moment to complete the following rating worksheet to assist with planning functional therapy for you.

Directions: Rate the importance of the following kinds of information.

Key: 1 = Important

2 = Moderately Important

3 = Not Important

UNDERSTANDING

____ a story someone relays at a party

____ an explanation given over the telephone

____ news reports

____ discussions with spouse, family member, or friend

____ radio talk shows

____ movies

____ interview questions

____ work-related information (e.g., instructions from supervisor, discussions with co-workers)

Please describe:

1. _____

2. _____

3. _____

____ academic-related information (e.g., lectures, discussions with classmates)

Please describe:

1. _____

2. _____

3. _____

____ other

Please describe:

1. _____

2. _____

3. _____

READING:

____ legal contracts

____ stock portfolios

____ novels or other leisure reading material

____ computer program instructions

____ mail and other correspondence

____ newspaper and magazines

____ work-related information (e.g., job manuals, professional materials and publications)

Please describe:

1. _____

2. _____

3. _____

____ academic-related information (e.g., course syllabus, textbooks)

Please describe:

1. _____

2. _____

3. _____

____ other

Please describe:

1. _____

2. _____

3. _____

INFORMATION PROCESSING TASK
PROCESSING FACTUAL INFORMATION

PURPOSE:

The purpose of this task is to improve the client's ability to process, integrate, recall, and apply higher level verbal or written factual information.

DIRECTIONS:

Present the client with either a factual video or audio cassette tape recording or reading passage and instruct him or her to read or listen to the information and then teach or explain it to the clinician in his or her own words.

Listening Examples: taped news segments, taped radio talk shows, taped class lectures, taped seminars

Reading Examples: magazine articles (e.g., *Time, U.S. News and World Report, Reader's Digest, Prevention*), stock prospectus, academic text chapters, contracts, leases, seminar information, professional journal articles, work-related articles

SUGGESTIONS FOR HIERARCHICAL PRESENTATION:

1. Begin presenting personally relevant and functional information at the sentence, paragraph, or multi-paragraph level, **gradually increasing the length**. As the client masters a certain length, repeat similar tasks at this level (same format and type of information) with **gradual increases in speed of presentation** (for verbal information) **or time limits** (for written information).

2. Utilize this task format and type of information (with several different listening or reading samples) to **teach and allow for practice** of compensatory listening, reading, and memory strategies to maximize success.

PRIMARY SKILLS TARGETED:

1. Auditory Information Processing and Comprehension
2. Visual Information Processing and Comprehension
3. Sustained Attention
4. Working Memory Capacity

TO ADDRESS THE RELATED SKILL OF:	INCORPORATE THIS TASK MODIFICATION:
1. Speed of Processing	For reading, impose time constraint, gradually reducing time allowed
	For listening, gradually increase speed of presentation
2. Selective Attention	Require client to complete task in a distracting environment (e.g., news talk radio, others talking in background, visual distractions)

3. Alternating Attention

Have client respond to interruptions from clinician and then resume reading

4. Divided Attention

Have client simultaneously listen and take notes

5. Written Expression

Have client explain information in writing

6. Memory

Have client explain information following a slight delay, after completing a different task, at the end of the session, or the following day

Develop or utilize compensatory memory strategies

PERFORMANCE MEASURES:

Evaluate the following:

- Percentage of presented facts included in explanation
- Percentage of presented details included in explanation
- Ability to integrate information for accurate and thorough comprehension and application
- Ability to clearly explain information (may indicate clarity of understanding as long as verbal or written skills are not significantly impaired)
- Effect of task modification(s) on performance (e.g., impact of attention and time issues when processing information with distractions or under time constraints)
- Ability to independently utilize compensatory memory strategies effectively

INFORMATION PROCESSING TASK
PROCESSING INSTRUCTIONAL INFORMATION

PURPOSE:

The purpose of this task is to improve the client's ability to process, integrate, recall, and apply higher level verbal or written instructional information.

DIRECTIONS:

Present the client with either an instructional video or audio cassette tape recording or reading passage and instruct him or her to read or listen to the information and then teach or explain it to the clinician in his or her own words.

Listening Examples: taped "how-to" news segments, taped radio talk shows, taped "how-to" magazine articles

Reading Examples: computer program manuals, product manuals for assembling, repair manuals, job manuals, "how-to" magazine or newspaper articles

SUGGESTIONS FOR HIERARCHICAL PRESENTATION:

1. Begin presenting personally relevant and functional information at the sentence, paragraph, or multi-paragraph level, **gradually increasing the length**. As the client masters a certain length, repeat similar tasks at this level (same format and type of information) with **gradual increases in speed of presentation** (for verbal information) **or time limits** (for written information).

2. Utilize this task format and type of information (with several different listening or reading samples) to **teach and allow for practice** of compensatory listening, reading, and memory strategies to maximize success.

PRIMARY SKILLS TARGETED:

1. Auditory Information Processing and Comprehension
2. Visual Information Processing and Comprehension
3. Sustained Attention
4. Working Memory Capacity

TO ADDRESS THE RELATED SKILL OF:	INCORPORATE THIS TASK MODIFICATION:
1. Speed of Processing	For reading, impose time constraint, gradually reducing time allowed
	For listening, gradually increase speed of presentation
2. Selective Attention	Require client to complete task in a distracting environment (e.g., news talk radio, others talking in background, visual distractions)

3. Alternating Attention	Have client respond to interruptions from clinician and then resume reading
4. Divided Attention	Have client simultaneously listen and take notes
5. Written Expression	Have client explain information in writing
6. Reasoning and Problem Solving	Have client actually follow presented instructions
7. Memory	Have client explain information following a slight delay, after completing a different task, at the end of the session, or the following day
	Develop or utilize compensatory memory strategies

PERFORMANCE MEASURES:

Evaluate the following:

- Percentage of presented facts included in explanation

- Percentage of presented details included in explanation

- Ability to integrate information for accurate and thorough comprehension and application

- Ability to clearly explain information (may indicate clarity of understanding as long as verbal or written skills are not significantly impaired)

- Effect of task modification(s) on performance (e.g., impact of attention and time issues when processing information with distractions and time constraints)

- Ability to independently utilize compensatory memory strategies effectively

INFORMATION PROCESSING TASK
PROCESSING NARRATIVE INFORMATION

PURPOSE:

The purpose of this task is to improve the client's ability to process, integrate, recall, and apply higher level verbal or written narrative information.

DIRECTIONS:

Present the client with either a narrative video or audio cassette tape recording or reading passage and instruct him or her to read or listen to the information and then teach or explain it to the clinician in his or her own words.

Listening Examples: taped *Reader's Digest* stories, stories presented on the radio, books on tape

Reading Examples: novel chapters, stories in magazines

SUGGESTIONS FOR HIERARCHICAL PRESENTATION:

1. Begin presenting personally relevant and functional information at the sentence, paragraph, or multi-paragraph level, **gradually increasing the length**. As the client masters a certain length, repeat similar tasks at this level (same format and type of information) with **gradual increases in speed of presentation** (for verbal information) **or time limits** (for written information).

2. Utilize this task format and type of information (with several different listening or reading samples) to **teach and allow for practice** of compensatory listening, reading, and memory strategies to maximize success.

PRIMARY SKILLS TARGETED:

1. Auditory Information Processing and Comprehension
2. Visual Information Processing and Comprehension
3. Sustained Attention
4. Working Memory Capacity

TO ADDRESS THE RELATED SKILL OF:	INCORPORATE THIS TASK MODIFICATION:
1. Speed of Processing	For reading, impose time constraint, gradually reducing time allowed
	For listening, gradually increase speed of presentation
2. Selective Attention	Require client to complete task in a distracting environment (e.g., news talk radio, others talking in background, visual distractions)

3. Alternating Attention   Have client respond to interruptions from clinician and then resume reading

4. Divided Attention   Have client simultaneously listen and take notes

5. Written Expression   Have client explain information in writing

6. Memory   Have client explain information following a slight delay, after completing a different task, at the end of the session, or the following day

Develop or utilize compensatory memory strategies

PERFORMANCE MEASURES:

Evaluate the following:

- Percentage of presented facts included in explanation
- Percentage of presented details included in explanation
- Ability to integrate information for accurate and thorough comprehension and application
- Ability to clearly explain information (may indicate clarity of understanding as long as verbal or written skills are not significantly impaired)
- Effect of task modification(s) on performance (e.g., impact of attention and time issues when processing information with distractions and time constraints)
- Ability to independently utilize compensatory memory strategies effectively

INFORMATION PROCESSING TASK
PROCESSING PERSUASIVE INFORMATION

PURPOSE:

The purpose of this task is to improve the client's ability to process, integrate, recall, and apply higher level verbal or written persuasive information.

DIRECTIONS:

Present the client with either a persuasive video or audio cassette tape recording or reading passage and instruct him or her to read or listen to the information and then teach or explain it to the clinician in his or her own words, including his or her opinion and decision.

Listening Examples: editorials on the news, taped debates, taped campaign speeches, taped sales pitches

Reading Examples: magazine articles (e.g., *Consumer Reports*), lengthy advertisements, newspaper editorials, product sales brochures

SUGGESTIONS FOR HIERARCHICAL PRESENTATION:

1. Begin presenting personally relevant and functional information at the sentence, paragraph, or multi-paragraph level, **gradually increasing the length**. As the client masters a certain length, repeat similar tasks at this level (same format and type of information) with **gradual increases in speed of presentation** (for verbal information) **or time limits** (for written information).

2. Utilize this task format and type of information (with several different listening or reading samples) to **teach and allow for practice** of compensatory listening, reading, and memory strategies to maximize success.

PRIMARY SKILLS TARGETED:

1. Auditory Information Processing and Comprehension
2. Visual Information Processing and Comprehension
3. Sustained Attention
4. Working Memory Capacity

TO ADDRESS THE RELATED SKILL OF:	INCORPORATE THIS TASK MODIFICATION:
1. Speed of Processing	For reading, impose time constraint, gradually reducing time allowed
	For listening, gradually increase speed of presentation
2. Selective Attention	Require client to complete task in a distracting environment (e.g., talk radio, others talking in background, visual distractions)

3. Alternating Attention	Have client respond to interruptions from clinician and then resume reading
4. Divided Attention	Have client simultaneously listen and take notes
5. Verbal Expression	Have client explain opinions, arguments, and decisions using newly learned facts
6. Written Expression	Have client explain information in writing
7. Reasoning and Problem Solving	Have client provide rationale for decision
8. Memory	Have client explain information following a slight delay, after completing a different task, at the end of the session, or the following day
	Develop or utilize compensatory memory strategies

PERFORMANCE MEASURES:

Evaluate the following:

- Percentage of presented facts included in explanation

- Percentage of presented details included in explanation

- Ability to integrate information for accurate and thorough comprehension and application

- Ability to clearly explain information (may indicate clarity of understanding as long as verbal or written skills are not significantly impaired)

- Ability to utilize reasoning skills to comprehend and explain an argument

- Effect of task modification(s) on performance (e.g., impact of attention and time issues when processing information with distractions and time constraints)

- Ability to independently utilize compensatory memory strategies effectively

INFORMATION PROCESSING TASK
PROS AND CONS OF AN ISSUE

PURPOSE:

The purpose of this task is to improve the client's ability to process, integrate, recall, and restate controversial information.

DIRECTIONS:

Present the client with either a controversial video or audio cassette tape recording or reading passage including two opposing opinions and justification for each, and instruct him or her to read or listen to the information and then restate the details and opinions for both sides of the issue to the clinician in his or her own words.

Listening Examples: taped political news segments, taped political debates, taped radio talk shows, taped seminars

Reading Examples: magazine articles (e.g., *Time, U.S. News and World Report, Consumer Reports*), newspaper editorials

SUGGESTIONS FOR HIERARCHICAL PRESENTATION:

1. Begin presenting personally relevant and functional information at the sentence, paragraph, or multi-paragraph level, **gradually increasing the length**. As the client masters a certain length, repeat similar tasks at this level (same format and type of information) with **gradual increases in speed** of presentation (for verbal information) **or time limits** (for written information).

2. Utilize this task format and type of information (with several different listening or reading samples) to **teach and allow for practice** of compensatory listening, reading, and memory strategies to maximize success.

PRIMARY SKILLS TARGETED:

1. Auditory Information Processing
2. Visual Information Processing
3. Sustained Attention
4. Reasoning
5. Retention and Recall
6. Thought Formulation, Organization, Elaboration

TO ADDRESS THE RELATED SKILL OF:	INCORPORATE THIS TASK MODIFICATION:
1. Speed of Processing	For reading, impose time constraint, gradually reducing time allowed
	For listening, gradually increase speed of presentation

2. Selective Attention

Require client to complete task in a distracting environment (e.g., news talk radio, others talking in background, visual distractions)

3. Alternating Attention

Have client respond to interruptions from clinician and then resume reading

4. Divided Attention

Have client simultaneously listen and take notes

5. Written Expression

Have client explain information in writing

6. Memory

Have client explain information following a slight delay, after completing a different task, at the end of the session, or the following day

Develop or utilize compensatory memory strategies

PERFORMANCE MEASURES:

Evaluate the following:

- Percentage of presented facts included in explanation

- Percentage of presented details included in explanation

- Level of integration of information for accurate and thorough comprehension

- Ability to clearly summarize and explain opinions and opposing issues

- Effect of task modification(s) on performance (e.g., time constraints, distractions)

- Ability to independently utilize compensatory memory strategies effectively

INFORMATION PROCESSING TASK
RESPONSE TO QUESTIONS

PURPOSE:

The purpose of this task is to improve the client's ability to process lengthy, written or verbal information for enhanced integration, recall, and retention.

DIRECTIONS:

Present the client with a lengthy article from a personally relevant magazine, such as *Reader's Digest*, and instruct the client to either read or listen to the article, and be prepared to answer related questions. Comprehension and recall will be assessed through the client's verbal responses to questions presented verbally by the clinician.

SUGGESTIONS FOR HIERARCHICAL PRESENTATION:

1. Begin presenting personally relevant and functional information at the sentence, paragraph, or multi-paragraph level, **gradually increasing the length**. As the client masters a certain length, repeat similar tasks at this level (same format and type of information) with **gradual increases in speed of presentation** (for verbal information) **or time limits** (for written information).

2. Utilize this task format and type of information (with several different listening or reading samples) to **teach and allow for practice** of compensatory listening, reading, and memory strategies to maximize success.

PRIMARY SKILLS TARGETED:

1. Auditory Information Processing and Comprehension
2. Visual Information Processing and Comprehension
3. Sustained Attention
4. Retention and Recall
5. Reasoning

TO ADDRESS THE RELATED SKILL OF:	INCORPORATE THIS TASK MODIFICATION:
1. Speed of Processing	For reading, impose time constraint, gradually reducing time allowed
	For listening, gradually increase speed of presentation
2. Selective Attention	Require client to complete task in a distracting environment (e.g., news talk radio, others talking in background, visually stimulating environment)

PERFORMANCE MEASURES:

Evaluate the following:

- Percentage of comprehension questions correct
- Effect of task modification(s) on performance (e.g., time constraints, distractions)
- Effective use of compensatory strategies

QUESTIONS

Utilize the following list of ideas to assist you in preparing questions pertaining to the specific article chosen by the clinician or client.

1. Provide three facts pertaining to the article.

2. Provide three opinions as stated in the article.

3. Provide three conclusions you have reached after reading or listening to this article.

4. Discuss your opinion as it relates to the author's point of view.

5. Provide a chronological sequence of events as they occurred in the article.

6. Briefly summarize the article in your own words, including at least five details.

7. How does the information from the article relate to your previous knowledge of this subject?

8. Did the article change your views regarding this topic? If yes, how?

9. Provide three pros and cons regarding the information presented.

10. What strategies did you utilize to assist you with processing, integrating, and recalling this information?

INFORMATION PROCESSING TASK
PROCESSING AND RETAINING DETAILS

PURPOSE:

The purpose of this task is to improve the client's ability to process, retain, and recall specific information (details) from information presented verbally or in writing.

DIRECTIONS:

Auditory: Verbally present information segments, encouraging the client to make notes of salient facts and details. Subsequent to an informative presentation, ask client to restate detailed information from notes.

Visual: Instruct client to read suggested information, making notes of salient facts and details. *(Clinician may review same reading material during this time for efficient time management, and develop outline of facts and details).* Following client's completion of the reading material, ask client to restate as many details as possible.

Listening Examples: clinician's verbal presentation of news segments or one-to-three page articles from client's personal or work-related interest magazines, audiotaped news presentation, instructional audiotapes, or videotapes

Reading Examples: client's personally relevant interest magazines, news and informational articles from popular magazines (e.g., *Reader's Digest, Consumer Reports, Time, Newsweek*), chapter sections from student texts

SUGGESTIONS FOR HIERARCHICAL PRESENTATION:

1. Begin presenting personally relevant and functional information at the sentence, paragraph, or multi-paragraph level, **gradually increasing the length**. As the client masters a certain length, repeat similar tasks at this level (same format and type of information) with **gradual increases in speed of presentation** (for verbal information) **or time limits** (for written information).

2. Utilize this task format and type of information (with many different listening or reading samples) to **teach and allow for practice** of compensatory listening, reading, and memory strategies to maximize success.

PRIMARY SKILLS TARGETED:

1. Auditory Information Processing and Comprehension
2. Visual Information Processing and Reading Comprehension
3. Sustained Attention
4. Divided Attention (listening or reading, and notetaking)
5. Working Memory

TO ADDRESS THE RELATED SKILL OF:	INCORPORATE THIS TASK MODIFICATION:
1. Selective Attention	Require client to complete task in a distracting environment (e.g., talk radio, others talking in background, visual distractions)
2. Long-Term Memory Recall	Without using notes as reference, have the client restate main ideas and five details during the following therapy session
	Develop or utilize compensatory memory strategies
3. Speed of Processing	Increase rate of clinician's verbal presentation

PERFORMANCE MEASURES:

Evaluate the following:

- Percentage of presented details included in client's recall of information

- Ability to use compensatory strategy of effective note-taking (key words, phrases) to aid information retention and recall

- Ability to process and integrate information to improve comprehension and recall in the verbal and written modalities

- Ability to process information at an increasing rate, length, and complexity in the verbal and written modalities

- Ability to retain and recall new information

- Ability to sustain attention during continuous auditory or visual task

- Effect of distractions on ability to process, retain, and recall details in both the verbal and written modalities

INFORMATION PROCESSING TASK
SUMMARIZING VERBAL AND WRITTEN INFORMATION

PURPOSE:

The purpose of this task is to improve the client's ability to process and retain details of information presented in the auditory or visual modality, and provide an organized verbal summary of the salient information.

DIRECTIONS:

Auditory: Verbally present information article, encouraging client to make notes using key words and phrases. Following clinician's verbal presentation, request client to develop verbal summary to present to clinician. *Client may need a brief amount of time to prepare summary comments.*

Visual: Instruct client to read suggested information, making notes of salient facts and details. Following client's completion of the reading material, ask client to present an organized verbal summary or formulate a cohesive written summary. *Client may need brief preparation time to organize thoughts.*

Listening Examples: clinician's verbal presentation or audiotape of lengthy news segments, one-to-three page articles from client's personal or work-related interest magazines, instructional audiotapes, or videotapes

Reading Examples: client's personally relevant interest magazines, professional journals, news and informational articles from popular magazines (e.g., *Reader's Digest, Consumer Reports, Time, Newsweek*), chapter sections from student text

SUGGESTIONS FOR HIERARCHICAL PRESENTATION:

1. Begin presenting personally relevant and functional information at the sentence, paragraph, or multi-paragraph level, **gradually increasing the length**. As the client masters a certain length, repeat similar tasks at this level (same format and type of information) with gradual increases in **speed of presentation** (for verbal information) **or time limits** (for written information).

2. Utilize this task format and type of information (with several different listening or reading samples) to **teach and allow for practice** of compensatory listening, reading, and memory strategies to maximize success.

PRIMARY SKILLS TARGETED:

1. Auditory Information Processing and Comprehension
2. Visual Information Processing and Reading Comprehension
3. Sustained Attention
4. Divided Attention (listening or reading, and notetaking)
5. Higher Level Word Retrieval

TO ADDRESS THE RELATED SKILL OF:	INCORPORATE THIS TASK MODIFICATION:
1. Speed of Processing	Increase rate of clinician's verbal presentation Impose time constraints during reading task
2. Selective Attention	Require client to complete task in a distracting environment (e.g., news talk radio, windows open in a noisy area, visual distractions)
3. Verbal or Written Thought	Have client summarize information (verbally or in writing) in an organized, concise manner
4. Memory Recall	Have client restate information (verbally or in writing), without referring to notes, to aid accurate recall

PERFORMANCE MEASURES:

Evaluate the following:

■ Ability to process information of increasing rate, length, and complexity in both the verbal and written modalities

■ Ability to process and integrate information to improve comprehension and recall

■ Ability to aid information processing, retention, and recall by use of effective note-taking (key words and phrases)

■ Ability to formulate thoughts and organize information for verbal presentation or written summary

■ Ability to rapidly access words to verbally summarize information

■ Effect of distractions on ability to retain and recall information

HOME PRACTICE TASKS

Several of the ideas listed below can be completed during the monitoring period of treatment, with the clinician recording client performance. Other ideas can be suggested to the client upon discharge to promote maintenance of therapy gains.

- Engage in discussions with family and friends regarding hobbies, current events, or topics of interest

- Call friends and discuss common topics

- Write letters to family and friends

- Make requests or complaints over the telephone to accurately discuss and obtain information

- Watch the evening news with a family member and discuss the topics and your related opinions

- Take an adult education class on a topic of personal interest to practice processing and learning new information

- Read and discuss daily mail to encourage processing of information and participation in family matters

- Read and discuss articles and books of interest with a friend or family member

- If available, utilize a computer for word processing and Internet communication

- Listen to a radio talk show and make notes or comments to yourself on the information you are hearing

- Actively attempt to learn two new pieces of information each day through listening

- Actively attempt to learn two new pieces of information each day through reading

SUGGESTIONS FOR FAMILIES

■ Provide verbal information in brief amounts or shorter units

■ Discuss verbal information at a normal or slowed rate (not necessarily louder) to allow for adequate processing and comprehension

■ Reassure family member that you will repeat detailed or lengthy information and provide clarification as needed

■ Encourage family member to paraphrase comments or ask questions to confirm accuracy of information

■ Include your family member in family discussions, such as when reviewing important financial or household matters; prompt each person to offer opinions

■ Cue family member to utilize compensatory strategies for enhanced processing of verbal or written information

■ Allow family member to complete tasks that require listening and reading skills

■ Encourage family member to discuss information he or she has read to enhance comprehension and integration

■ Reduce the amount of external distractions (e.g., radio, television) to enhance effective communication

■ Display patience and understanding

CHAPTER 8

Treating Executive Functioning Impairments

DEFINITION

Executive Functioning

The cognitive language skill that incorporates the higher level skills of self-awareness, self-monitoring, goal-setting, planning, initiation, inhibition, task completion, cognitive flexibility, response to therapeutic feedback, and goal-directed behavior. According to Mateer (1987), executive functions "organize and regulate behavior necessary for accomplishment" (p. 1).

Specific to the mild-to-moderate TBI population, impairments in this skill area may manifest themselves in difficulties such as:

- Reduced deficit awareness and insight regarding impact of deficits on daily demands, family relationships, and work responsibilities

- Difficulty determining and selecting personal goals or setting priorities

- Limited ability to sequence steps of a task or follow complex and lengthy directions

- Decreased task initiation and execution to begin or complete daily living, school, or work-related tasks

- Difficulty planning a schedule or keeping appointments

- Decreased ability to monitor or inhibit inappropriate behavioral or emotional responses

- Compromised response to constructive feedback in order to modify behavior or adjust task approach

- Limited ability to consider alternative reactions, approaches, or plans to successfully complete complex tasks or appropriately interact with others

- Reduced ability to monitor time and efficiently complete tasks in a timely manner

- Limited self-monitoring skills necessary for error detection and correction to ensure accurate task completion

OTHER CONTRIBUTING COGNITIVE IMPAIRMENTS

The following are cognitive impairments that may be seen in individuals with mild-to-moderate TBI and may contribute to executive dysfunction:

Difficulties with:	May lead to:
1. Attention/Concentration	Difficulty processing, concentrating, responding to constructive feedback to make needed changes
	Reduced attention to behavior and task performance necessary for successful self-monitoring
	Limited ability to sustain attention in order to initiate, plan, and complete a task
	Reduced alternating and divided attention required for completion of complex or multiple tasks

	Sensory overload, which interferes with management of information necessary to plan and complete tasks
2. Organization	Difficulty generating an organized plan for task initiation and completion
	Difficulty processing and organizing information to integrate task instructions and demands necessary for task completion
	Difficulty organizing time, schedules, and plans
3. Cognitive Flexibility	Reduced ability to create a variety of plans for task completion or to approach task in an alternative manner
4. Speed of Information Processing	Delayed initiation of plan due to compromised understanding of complex instructions
	Interrupted task completion due to difficulty with comprehending rapidly presented resource information
5. Memory	Difficulty retaining and recalling detailed information to accurately complete tasks
6. Reasoning	Difficulty comprehending, reasoning, and integrating new information to solve problems and make decisions

FUNCTIONAL IMPLICATIONS OF
EXECUTIVE FUNCTIONING IMPAIRMENTS

The following is a list of many of the abilities needed for successful functioning in the natural environments of home, work, and school. Impairments in executive functioning in people with mild-to-moderate TBI may compromise performance in these functional environments. You are encouraged to explore these and other related activities with your clients to create functional and personally relevant therapy tasks and to maximize carry-over of therapeutic gains to the natural environment. As executive functioning deficits can impact the initiation and completion of the majority of daily living, school, and work tasks, only a sampling of examples has been provided to promote a clearer understanding of the functional impact of such deficits. These examples may stimulate additional ideas that are more personally relevant to your individual client.

In the Home

Ability to...

■ **Initiate and complete daily living and household activities in a timely manner**

Examples:

Maintain home cleanliness and organization (daily and weekly cleaning schedule)

List and complete daily errands

Plan and prepare family meals

Maintain laundry schedule

Schedule family appointments and activities

Manage timely arrival at planned activities

Complete bill paying and banking on a timely basis

Organize and prepare daily items for self and others, if needed

Return telephone calls and relay messages to others

Monitor and document amount of time needed to complete each task

■ **Display flexibility and assess task planning and completion**

Examples:

Self-monitor ability to successfully complete tasks and activities on a timely basis

Prioritize daily tasks and family needs

Modify planned activities according to time schedule

Organize a list of tasks not completed for the next day's schedule

Set realistic goals for accomplishing tasks and activities based on completion time and priority list

At Work

Ability to...

■ **Initiate and complete work-related tasks and job responsibilities in a timely manner**

Examples:

Maintain awareness of daily and weekly job tasks

Organize and sequence priority tasks according to time demands

List and complete steps of job tasks to facilitate timely completion

Prepare written lists and memos of important information to share with coworkers

Monitor and document amount of time needed to complete each task

Maintain an organized system of notes for instructions from supervisor and dates for task completion

■ **Display flexibility and assess task planning and completion**

Examples:

Prioritize daily work tasks and job demands

Self-monitor ability to successfully complete tasks and activities on a timely basis

Modify planned tasks according to time schedule

Organize a list of tasks not completed for the next day's schedule

Set realistic goals for accomplishing tasks based on completion time and priority list

At School

Ability to...

■ **Initiate and complete academic assignments in a timely manner**

Examples:

Maintain awareness of course assignments and examination schedules; document in datebook

Organize notebooks for lecture notes and textbook notes

List questions to clarify information and better understand concepts

Prepare daily schedule of classes, work schedule, social activities, and other time demands; schedule time blocks needed to include transportation time, study time, etc.

Develop a consistent weekly study schedule to review lecture notes, complete readings, and prepare for exams

■ **Display flexibility and assess assignment planning and completion**

Examples:

Prioritize daily school assignments and educational demands

Self-monitor ability to successfully complete assignments on a timely basis

Modify planned assignments according to time schedule

Organize a list of assignments not completed for the next day's schedule

Set realistic goals for accomplishing school tasks based on completion time and priority list

In addition to the executive functioning tasks provided in the following pages, you may utilize the information listed above to create unique therapy tasks that will be most meaningful for your client, depending on his or her goal environment. Please refer to the cover sheet describing the skill impairment to assist you with addressing related skills simultaneously.

COMPENSATORY STRATEGIES

Select from this list the executive functioning strategies that would be most helpful to and effectively utilized by your clients, considering their skill limitations and potential home, work, and school environments. It is recommended that these strategies be taught to the client and incorporated into the therapy sessions until the client is able to utilize them successfully and independently. Additionally, allow for practice of the specific strategy in the target environment to ensure successful carryover.

- Write out goals and plans for the day, week, month, and year for the home, work, and school environments (Goal Setting, Planning)

- Each morning, read your list of plans for the day (leave in a conspicuous place and write at the top "NEED TO COMPLETE TODAY") (Initiation)

- Create a daily checklist with two headings: "What I need to complete today" and "What I need to get started" (Initiation)

- Plan tasks and activities to accomplish during optimal times to enhance efficient and successful completion (peak energy times, minimal distractions, time available) (Planning)

- Place notes around the home or work environment to remind you to use compensatory strategies (e.g., "Check your datebook") (Task completion)

- Utilize schedules, a beeping watch, a timer, or small note saying "check the time" (Time sense)

- Allow yourself extra time for tasks you view as challenging or time consuming (Time sense)

- Prior to working on a task, organize all the materials you will need and place them at your work space; use a task checklist to make sure all materials are readily accessible; sequence steps to the task, determine amount of time needed for each step, and check off each step as completed (Goal setting, Planning, Task completion)

- While working on a task, place a note within your view that states "How am I doing with this task? Recheck my work" (Self-monitoring)

- Try to get into the habit of always asking yourself "How am I doing on this task?" Then check! (Self-monitoring)

- Periodically review a list of your functional limitations, as well as therapy goals, skill improvements, and helpful changes in your life (Awareness)

EXECUTIVE FUNCTIONING TASK
VARIOUS TASKS AND ACTIVITIES TO PLAN, INITIATE, AND COMPLETE

PURPOSE:

The purpose of the activities included under this skill area is to improve the client's ability to plan, initiate, organize, and complete tasks on a weekly basis.

DIRECTIONS:

To promote task planning, initiation, organization, time management, task completion, and self-monitoring, initially have your client choose a complex task to complete in therapy with your guidance (see list of task ideas on the following page or create your own). Following your client's demonstration of improved executive functioning skills, instruct your client to choose one activity from the list of task ideas to complete each week outside of the therapy setting without your guidance. Using the Client Worksheet and Questionnaire, as well as the Clinician Task Documentation sheet, assess the client's ability to complete each task successfully and on a timely basis.

POSSIBLE TASKS AND ACTIVITIES

Tasks to complete in therapy:

- Review, sort, file, or discard collected mail or magazines (have client bring to session)

- Schedule and generate responses to requested information, complete required forms, and discuss follow-up action regarding important matters (identified by reviewing mail)

- Review new recipes and organize a shopping list to prepare a full-course meal (brunch, dinner, barbecue) for family or friends (six people minimum)

- Prepare a list of items needed and create a personalized gift for someone special

- Create personal file cards for family members, friends, and close associates, with important information such as names of spouse, children, contact numbers, birthdates, and anniversaries, in order to acknowledge significant dates and events with a call or card

- Review mail catalogs to locate specific, hard-to-find items, as requested by clinician, and provide all necessary ordering information

- Create a vehicle checklist for maintenance and repairs, and complete it with current information

- Develop a household monthly budget form to document and track fixed and variable weekly and monthly expenses

- Investigate five new, interesting restaurants of your choice by obtaining information regarding food variety, price range, appropriate attire, handicapped accessibility, and location

- Using a newspaper, learn and present information on three possible job prospects or volunteer positions of interest

Tasks to complete at home:

- Determine a household task that needs to be done, list and obtain items needed to accomplish the task, and schedule when to complete it

- Comparison shop at three locations for a specific item to determine the best purchase price

- At a library or bookstore, locate a book on a specified topic of interest, read it, and prepare a brief summary of information

- Volunteer to be a group leader (at school or work), determine a group project, and prepare an initial outline of what needs to be accomplished

- Locate travel brochures and determine two possible locations for your next vacation; identify pros and cons (travel time, travel and hotel costs, weather, etc.) of those particular destinations

- Obtain a local bus schedule and contact a taxi service to determine possible means of transportation to therapy, a volunteer position, or your work, and document the available times and transportation costs

■ Contact three banks and obtain information regarding their interest percentage for savings accounts and their service charges for checking accounts and automatic teller machines

■ Reorganize your garage and work area to itemize tools and equipment and make a list of needed items for home repairs

CLIENT TASK WORKSHEET

(may be completed with clinician or independently)

CLIENT NAME: _____ WEEK/YEAR: _____

TASK OR ACTIVITY CHOSEN TO COMPLETE: _____

_____

DATE PLANNED TO COMPLETE: _____ ACTUAL DATE COMPLETED: _____

I. What steps need to be completed to accomplish this task?

1.   6.

2   7.

3.   8.

4.   9.

5.   10.

2. What items need to be organized or purchased to complete this task?

1.	6.
2	7.
3.	8.
4.	9.
5.	10.

3. Who should you contact or where should you go to obtain needed information?

4. How much time do you estimate you will need to complete the entire task or activity? If possible, break down the time needed for each step.

5. What strategies will you use to assist you?

CLIENT FOLLOW-UP QUESTIONNAIRE

1. Were you able to complete the task?

2. Was it completed on time?

3. What difficulties did you encounter when attempting to accomplish this task or activity?

4. What, if any, assistance did you need from others?

5. What strategies did you use to assist you in completing this task or activity?

6. What went smoothly to enhance your self-confidence while you were completing this task or activity?

7. If you were unable to complete the task as planned, what alternative steps could have been taken or what other possible arrangements could have been made?

8. Are there any other related tasks or activities you would like to attempt in the future?

CLINICIAN TASK DOCUMENTATION

CLIENT NAME: _____ WEEK/YEAR: _____

TASK OR ACTIVITY CHOSEN TO COMPLETE: _____

_____

DATE PLANNED TO COMPLETE: _____ ACTUAL DATE COMPLETED: _____

Use the following rating scale to determine the client's ability to utilize various executive functioning skills to successfully complete assigned complex daily living tasks. Circle the level of assistance required under each statement below. When assistance was required, please describe specifically under "Comments." Assessment may be based on either the client's reporting or your observation of the task completion, which you may indicate by circling "R" or "O."

1 = no assistance needed   R = reported by client

2 = completed with assistance   O = observed by clinician

3 = unable to complete

R   O   **1.** Ability to understand the task instructions   1   2   3
COMMENTS:

R   O   **2.** Ability to determine the task or activity to be completed   1   2   3
COMMENTS:

R   O   **3.** Ability to sequence steps of the task   1   2   3
COMMENTS:

R   O   **4.** Ability to organize materials needed to complete the task   1   2   3
COMMENTS:

R   O   **5.** Ability to initiate the task or activity in a timely manner   1 2 3

           COMMENTS:

R   O   **6.** Ability to obtain needed resource information   1 2 3

           COMMENTS:

R   O   **7.** Ability to estimate time needed to complete the task or activity   1 2 3

           COMMENTS:

R   O   **8.** Ability to identify problems and determine alternative methods to accomplish the task or activity   1 2 3

           COMMENTS:

R   O   **9.** Ability to select and use compensatory strategies   1 2 3

           COMMENTS:

R   O   **10.** Ability to complete task or activity within specified time or within a reasonable time frame   1 2 3

           COMMENTS:

Did client report difficulty with associated skill impairments of:

____ Functional Memory

____ Information Processing

____ Concentration and Complex Attention Skills

____ Verbal or Written Expression

____ Reasoning/Problem Solving

COMMENTS:

Discuss with the client what skill limitations made accomplishing the task more difficult.

Discuss with the client what skill strengths assisted in task or activity completion.

HOME PRACTICE TASKS

Several of the ideas listed below can be completed during the monitoring period of treatment, with the clinician recording client performance. Other ideas can be suggested to the client on discharge to promote maintenance of therapy gains.

- Utilize daily personal tasks such as letter writing and bill paying to monitor your work (initiation and completion of tasks)

- Volunteer to plan and organize events for your family (e.g., party, family gathering, potluck dinner)

- Each day, set one goal for yourself and, at the end of the day, evaluate its completion

- Coordinate a daily and weekly schedule for yourself or a family member, based on a list of "to-do's"

- Organize a day or night out with a family member (spouse, child, sibling) or friend; schedule time and make arrangements for dinner, shopping, movie, coffee, etc.

- To enhance your time sense, practice estimating how long you think a task will take, then record the time when you begin and finish the task, and compare it to your estimate

- Coordinate a monthly or yearly calendar of important events (such as birthdays and anniversaries of family and friends) and check at the beginning of each month to send cards

- Develop a scavenger hunt for children or a road rally for adults, with items and locations

- Plan and complete a home improvement task; visualize the end result, and then generate a list of materials needed, purchase the items, sequence the steps, and execute the plan to complete the task.

- Attempt to reorganize one of the following: pantry, garage, basement, closet, kitchen drawer, dresser drawer, or attic and monitor your ability to plan and execute an organizational system

- Reward yourself on task completion by doing something enjoyable (taking a walk, watching a video, visiting a friend)

SUGGESTIONS FOR FAMILIES

- Provide your family member with verbal cues regarding time (e.g., "You have about 30 minutes to get ready")

- Remind your family member to set his or her watch, alarm, buzzer

- Expect that your family member may lose track of time and be late, so demonstrate patience

- Realize that your family member's inactivity may be due to an initiation problem rather than laziness or a lack of motivation

- Inquire about therapy, skill areas addressed, and improvements

- Inquire about the compensatory strategies your family member uses and which work best; attempt to monitor his or her use of strategies

- If needed, provide verbal reminders to utilize specific strategies for various skill limitations and tasks

- Consistently ask, "Did you recheck your work?" or "Now that you have finished, what do you need to do?" to promote self-monitoring as a habit

- Ask, "What are your plans for today?" (Begin first by stating your plans for the day as a model.)

- At the end of the day, ask your family member, "Did you complete or achieve what you wanted to today?" Discuss what was or was not completed

- Discuss what should be on tomorrow's list of things to do

CHAPTER 9

Therapy Documentation, Transition, and Discharge

THE USEFULNESS OF QUALITY THERAPY DOCUMENTATION

Clear and complete documentation of a client's performance on tasks presented in therapy is essential. Documentation fulfills a variety of purposes. First, it assists the clinician in knowing how to modify task complexity to ensure both success and challenge. Second, it provides the clinician with objective information regarding the client's skill improvement on specific tasks and how this corresponds with carryover of skill enhancement to actual daily functioning. It is important to be aware that, "performance variability is not a problem with all populations and is much more characteristic of individuals who have neurologic impairment, than of those who do not" (LaPointe, 1991, p. 6). Therefore, it is important to interpret performance variability on repeated tasks within and across daily sessions with caution. Overall, it would be more accurate and objective to consider improvement over weeks and months. Third, the clinician obtains objective data, which are useful when requesting additional treatment sessions or recommending discontinuation of services based on performance. Fourth, the information facilitates a more detailed, accurate therapy progress report and allows for comparison of the client's performance over time and across skill areas, as well as a more in-depth analysis of all skills needed to complete a task. For example, on an information processing task, careful and thorough documentation of performance may reveal a limitation in speed of processing rather than accuracy. From this information, more creative and individualized therapy tasks that specifically target a "subskill" limitation (e.g., speed), can be developed. Lastly, with clear and detailed documentation, the clinician is better prepared when consulted by other professionals, such as a vocational counselor, and when questioned about a client's abilities. Documentation is particularly useful when it pertains to tasks that simulate potential return-to-work duties.

DOCUMENTING TASK PERFORMANCE FOR TASKS IN THIS MANUAL

For most therapy tasks, there are multiple ways to monitor and interpret performance. For example, on a word-retrieval task, one clinician may monitor speed, while another clinician may monitor response creativity. Yet another may document both. Since components of performance to be documented vary depending on the client's skill strengths and limitations, therapy goals, and the desired outcome setting, we have provided performance measures for each of the therapy tasks in this manual. The clinician may choose several or all aspects of the task to document. Several of the measures are objective and allow tracking of performance using a number or percentage; others are more subjective and can only be documented narratively, using descriptive terms. Both types of information are highly beneficial for fulfilling the purposes of clear, detailed documentation as described above. The measures we have included encourage the clinician to monitor closely, document precisely, and describe thoroughly, a client's performance on the presented task, as well as on a task when it is modified in length or complexity.

TRANSITION AND DISCHARGE FROM THERAPY

As therapy goals are met, decisions must be made regarding a transition and discharge from formal treatment. In most cases, a gradual reduction is recommended to the point that a client may be seen once a month. Subsequently, monitoring through a monthly clinical visit or telephone call for approximately 3 months is a method of providing the client with clinical support and feedback as he or she assumes his or her preinjury or new responsibilities. In the case where a transition to a work or school setting is being coordinated, it is recommended that the clinican continue providing therapy on a reduced basis until a transition to the outcome setting is secured. It is then the role of the clinician to ensure carryover of improved cognitive-language skills to the work or school setting. At this point, the clinician's involvement should be reduced on a gradual basis, eventually to a monthly telephone call to the client for 3 months, for monitoring purposes. Prior to discharge, it is helpful to administer a re-evaluation to document skill gains, persisting skill limitations, and successful level of functioning. It is essential that the same tests and conditions used during the initial evaluation be utilized to ensure accurate skill comparisons.

FOLLOW-UP

In addition to the monthly monitoring calls, it is recommended that the clinician re-evaluate the client approximately 6 months following discharge to ensure maintenance of skill gains, and successful functioning in the natural outcome setting (e.g., home, work, school). Again, it is essential that the clinician utilize the same evaluation measures and conditions that were used on discharge for accurate comparison. Additionally, it is important to note whether the client was able to maintain successful, productive functioning in the natural outcome environment, 6 months later. Lastly, if the client has not successfully applied and maintained his or her improved skills in the natural environment, a brief reinitiation of therapy or a change in the established outcome setting may be warranted, and insurance approval may be necessary. If the client appears to be functioning successfully, the clinician's services are no longer required; however, the client should be encouraged to call with any future questions or concerns regarding his or her cognitive-language skills and how they impact his or her ability to return to his or her highest level of functioning.

APPENDIX 9-A

Sample Re-evaluation

CLIENT: Karen O'Conner
DATE OF BIRTH: November 25, 1935
DATE OF INJURY: December 10, 1994
DATE OF INITIAL EVALUATION: April 19 & 26, 1995
DATE OF RE-EVALUATION AND DISCHARGE: May 13 & 15, 1996

COGNITIVE-LANGUAGE THERAPY AND DISCHARGE SUMMARY

Karen O'Conner received individual cognitive-language therapy 4 to 6 hours per week for the past year. As Karen appears to have reached maximum benefit from therapeutic intervention and has attained both therapeutic and personal goals to the best of her ability, therapy was discontinued this month. Karen reported being pleased with her improved functioning and is aware of her remaining skill limitations. She is now comfortable in how to best compensate for residual limitations and is more accepting of them. In preparation for discharge from formal therapy this month, evaluation tests were readministered to objectively measure skill improvements and determine persisting limitations. In addition to functional gains in a variety of cognitive-language skill areas as reported by Karen and demonstrated in daily functioning, improvements were documented on a variety of objective assessment measures. The results are as follows:

Verbal Expression

While discussing her opinion on various topical and controversial issues, Karen demonstrated improved thought organization and expression, with no stuttering noted during this assessment. Higher level word-retrieval difficulties remained, however, on a much less interfering or noticeable basis. Karen was much less tangential and did not lose her train of thought, which had been observed during the initial evaluation. Improved word-retrieval and verbal expression skills were displayed on a variety of formal measures.

Test of Adolescent/Adult Word Finding (German, 1990)
Naming Subtest: Name pictures as fast as possible

	Pretherapy	*Post-therapy*
# named correctly:	92%	97%
% of words stuttered:	32%	0%

Scales of Cognitive Ability for Traumatic Brain Injury (Adamovich & Henderson, 1992)
Recall Subtest: Generate words beginning with target letter in 60 seconds

	Pretherapy	*Post-therapy*
# of words:	average: 12	average: 14
	(norm = 14+)	(norm = 14+)

During therapy sessions, Karen was provided with several compensatory strategies to assist her in clear, organized verbal expression during particularly challenging situations, such as while on the telephone with strangers. She is aware that her periodic word-retrieval difficulty and mild stuttering during moments of anxiety may not fully resolve. Still, her improved communication skills allow her to function independently.

Auditory Processing and Comprehension

Karen demonstrated improvements on a variety of auditory processing tests involving processing and retention of verbal directions, although her speed of processing and retention of details remains reduced for lengthy instructions.

Detroit Test of Learning Aptitude—2 (Hammill, 1985)
Oral Directions Subtest: Process, retain, and execute lengthy, complex directions, incorporating visual and motoric modalities

Pretherapy	*Post-therapy*
59%	74%

Executing Detailed Contingent Commands (nonstandardized)
"If *x* is true, then do this; if it isn't true, then do this."

Pretherapy	*Post-therapy*
63%	81%
with repetition: 75%	with repetition: 94%

Karen demonstrated improved auditory attention, processing, and retention for brief, paragraph length information. More functional, lengthy information remains challenging as Karen's speed of processing and integration of information continue to be reduced. Attention skills, compensatory strategies, and structured practice focusing on main ideas of verbal information were targeted in therapy and have enhanced Karen's ability to function more independently or compensate when necessary.

Memory and Learning

Karen has demonstrated significant improvement in her functional memory skills due to improved attention, increased organization, and effective use of compensatory strategies, as indicated by increased independence and productivity at home, as well as performance on the following objective tests:

Wechsler Memory Scale (Wechsler, 1945)
Associate Learning Subtest: Recall 10 word pairs with both high and low association, presented across three different trials

	Pretherapy	*Post-therapy*
Overall score:	10.5	16.5
	(mean = 11.94; s.d. = 4.53)	(mean = 11.94; s.d. = 4.53)

California Verbal Learning Test (Delis, Kramer, Kaplan, & Ober, 1987)
Recall, retain, and recognize a list of 16 words in four semantic cate-

gories, presented across five trials and following a time delay, as well as a distraction word list

Pretherapy	List A Trial 1	List A Trial 5	List B Distractor	Long Delay Free Recall	Long Delay Cued Recall
Raw Score:	5/16	10/16	4/16	8/16	10/16
Standard Score: (mean = 0; s.d. = 1)	-1	-1	-2	-1	-1
Percentage recalled	31%	63%	25%	50%	63%
Post-therapy					
Raw Score:	10/16	14/16	9/16	11/16	16/16
Standard Score: (mean = 0; s.d. = 1)	+1	+1	+1	0	+2
Percentage recalled	63%	88%	56%	69%	100%

Scales of Cognitive Ability for Traumatic Brain Injury (Adamovich & Henderson, 1992)
Recall Subtest: Visual and auditory tasks; word, sentence, and paragraph level

	Pretherapy	Post-therapy
Standard Score:	113	133
Percentile Rank:	81st	99th

Prospective Memory Screening (Sohlberg & Mateer, 1989)
Ability to initiate and carry out planned actions at designated times

	Pretherapy	Post-therapy
Total Score (out of 7)	3 (impaired)	5 (borderline impaired)

Overall, performance on various assessment measures of memory support Karen's reported improved memory functioning. Reduced performance on one test reflects a persisting attention or memory limitation that Karen will regularly need to take into consideration in her daily functioning. Fatigue and physical pain level clearly impact her attention and, therefore, functional memory skills. Yet, with this awareness, as well as consistent use of learned compensatory strategies, her functional memory skills are much improved.

Speed of Processing

Speed and Capacity of Language-Processing Test (Baddeley et al., 1992)
Read basic sentences as quickly as possible and determine if they make sense

	Pretherapy	*Post-therapy*
# Completed in 2 min.	31	56
# of errors	1	1
Scaled Score	6	10
Percentile Rank	<1st	50th

Although significant gains were made in Karen's speed of processing written information, current performance on this test, as well as on auditory processing tests, suggests a persisting generalized reduced speed of processing information (in reading, listening, and speaking modalities). Therefore, Karen will consistently need to compensate for this skill reduction by requesting repetition of information, focusing on key points, allowing for extra processing time, taking brief notes, using key cue words, or restating information for clarification.

Reasoning and Problem Solving

Scales of Cognitive Ability for Traumatic Brain Injury (Adamovich & Henderson, 1992)
Reasoning Subtest: Measure of basic reasoning skills

	Pretherapy	*Post-therapy*
Standard Score:	121	134
Percentile Rank:	92nd	99th
Severity:	Borderline Normal	Normal

Performance indicates improvement in Karen's ability to organize, analyze, and integrate detailed information in order to solve problems and make decisions. This improvement has been transferred to her own life and has significantly enhanced her confidence in making decisions, thereby increasing her level of independence and productivity at home.

Reading

Gray Oral Reading Tests—Revised (Wiederholt & Bryant, 1986)
Read paragraphs of 8 to 13 lines and respond to multiple choice factual and inferential questions without referring back to the paragraph

	Pretherapy	*Post-therapy*
Range of Response Accuracy:	60-80%	80-100%
Average Response Accuracy:	70%	83%

Executing Detailed Contingent Commands (nonstandardized)
"If *x* is true, then do this; if it isn't true, then do this."

Pretherapy	*Post-therapy*
94%	94%

Improvements on objective testing support Karen's reports of improved reading comprehension. She continues to experience reduced retention of information and will always benefit from rereading and taking notes on complex, lengthy information needed for future reference.

Writing

Functional writing skills were informally reassessed through a variety of writing tasks. When required to summarize page-length information in a paragraph, improved thought organization and clarity were displayed, although time delays and rewriting indicated persisting reduced thought formulation skills. When required to generate four sentences related to a topic sentence and use them to formulate a cohesive paragraph, Karen improved in her ability to form an integrated, organized paragraph through the use of transitions, specific examples, and clear sentence structure. Although writing was not directly targeted in therapy, it appears that improvements in processing, organization, and integration skills in the reading, speaking, and listening modalities have transferred to the writing modality.

Math

Kaufman Test of Educational Achievement (Kaufman & Kaufman, 1985) Math Computation Subtest: Ability to compute single, double, and triple digit problems, as well as fraction, decimal, and percentage problems involving addition, subtraction, multiplication, and division

	Pretherapy	*Post-therapy*
Computation Skills:	73%	80%

An improvement in Karen's knowledge of how to solve presented problems was displayed; however, reduced attention to details resulted in minor errors and, therefore, a minimal change in overall score. Yet, on the following test in which she was required to apply math knowledge and reasoning skills, basic computation and attention to details were much improved. The results are as follows:

Math Word Problems (nonstandardized)
Listen to brief word problems, write key information, and then apply math and reasoning skills to compute equations

	Pretherapy	*Post-therapy*
Reasoning and Sequencing Skills (Application)	92% accuracy	100% accuracy
Computation and Attention to Details	42% accuracy	92% accuracy

Summary and Recommendations

In summary, Karen demonstrated improvements in the treatment goal areas of verbal expression, auditory comprehension and retention, memory skills, complex attention (sustained, alternating, selective, and divided), speed of processing, reasoning and problem solving, organization, reading comprehension, writing, and functional math. Skill improvements were documented on objective testing, as well as noticed by Karen in her daily functioning. Skill limitations persist in the areas of: higher level word retrieval, integration and retention of lengthy verbal and written information, speed of processing, sustained attention, and functional memory. Additionally, cognitive-language functioning continues to become compromised during instances of stress, fatigue, and sensory overload. As stated earlier, Karen appears to have reached maximum benefit from therapeutic intervention and has attained both therapeutic and personal goals to the best of her ability. She is returning to her previous employment setting on a gradual basis. Therefore, it is recommended that she be discharged from individual therapy. Karen reported being pleased with her improved functioning and is aware of her persisting skill limitations and how to best compensate and accept them. Compensatory strategies learned in therapy were reviewed with Karen, and suggestions were provided to promote continued cognitive-language stimulation and maintenance of skill gains. Karen was encouraged to call this clinician should she notice a significant decline in her cognitive and communicative functioning. A re-evaluation will be scheduled in the next 3 to 6 months, to ensure that Karen has maintained her rehabilitation gains, independent of direct therapeutic intervention. It has truly been a pleasure working with such a motivated, conscientious, and determined individual who was strongly invested in her own rehabilitation. Karen's significant progress is an indication of the immense effort she put forth in every therapy session. Thank you for the opportunity to assist her and thank you for your support of our therapeutic services. If you have any questions, please do not hesitate to call.

Sincerely,

Mara B. Goodson M.A. CCC
Speech-Language Pathologist

References

Acimovic, M., Keatley, M., & Lemmon, J. (1993). The importance of qualitative indicators in the assessment of mild brain injury. *The Journal of Cognitive Rehabilitation, 11*(6), 8–14.

Americans with Disabilites Act of 1990, Public Law 101-476. 20 U.S.C. §§ 1400–1485.

American Psychiatric Association. (1994). *Diagnostic and statistical manual of mental disorders* (4th ed.) Washington DC: American Psychiatric Association.

Bennett, T. (1992). Conceptualizing traumatic brain injuries. *The Journal of Head Injury, 3*(1), 21–28.

Depoy, E. (1992). A comparison of standardized and observational assessment. *The Journal of Cognitive Rehabilitation, 10*(1), 30–32.

Fahy, J. F., & Schmitter, M. E. (1991). Current issues in memory research: What is prospective memory? *The Journal of Head Injury, 2*(4), 38–41.

Frank, E. M., & Barrineau, S. (1996). Current speech-language assessment protocols for adults with traumatic brain injury. *Journal of Medical Speech-Language Pathology, 4*(2), 81–101.

Hambacher, W. (1995). In J. Gelman. Preparing to take the stand as an expert witness. *Advance for Speech-Language Pathologists and Audiologists, 5*(49), 10–11, 24.

Kay, T. (1986). *Minor head injury: An introduction for professionals* (pp. 1–12). Washington DC: Brain Injury Association, Inc.

Kay, T. (1993). Neuropsychological treatment of mild traumatic brain injury. *The Journal of Head Trauma Rehabilitation, 8*(3), 74–85.

Kay, T., Harrington, D. E., Adams, R., Anderson, T., Berrol, S.,Cicerone, K., Dahlberg, C., Gerber, D., Goka, R., Harley, P., Hilt, J., Horn, L., Lehmkuhl, D., & Malec, J. (1993). Definition of mild traumatic brain injury. *The Journal of Head Trauma Rehabilitation, 8*(3), 86–87.

Kay, T., & Silver, S. M. (1988). The contribution of the neuropsychological evaluation to the vocational rehabilitation of the head-injured adult. *The Journal of Head Trauma Rehabilitation, 3*(1), 65–76.

Kraus, J., & McArthur, D. L. (1995). Epidemiology of brain injury. Los Angeles: University of California Los Angeles, Department of Epidemiology, Southern California Injury Prevention Research Center.

Kraus, J. F., & Nourjah, P. (1989). The epidemiology of mild head injury. In H. S. Levin, H. M. Eisenberg, & A. L. Benton (Eds.), *Mild head injury* (pp. 8–22). New York: Oxford University Press.

Kraus, J., & Sorenson, S. (1994). Epidemiology. In J. Silver,S. Yudofsky, & R. Hales (Eds.), *Neuropsychiatry of traumatic brain injury* (pp. 3–41). Washington DC: American Psychiatric Press.

LaPointe, L. (1991). *Base 10 Response Form* (Rev. Manual). San Diego, CA: Singular Publishing Group.

Lewkowicz, S. S., & Whitton, J. L. (1995). A new inventory for exploring neuropsychological change resulting from brain injury. *The Journal of Cognitive Rehabilitation, 13*(1), 8–20.

Mateer, C. (1987). Frontal lobe injury. [Bulletin]. Puyallup, WA: Good Samaritan Hospital, Center for Cognitive Rehabilitation.

Mateer, C., & Moore-Sohlberg, M. (1992, September). *Current perspectives in cognitive rehabilitation.* Presented at conference entitled

"Speaking of Cognition . . . Assessment and Intervention Strategies." Sponsored by Rehabilitation Services Midwest Medical Center, Indianapolis, IN.

McAllister, T. W. (1994). Mild traumatic brain injury and the postconcusive syndrome. In J. Silver, S. Yudofsky, & R. Hales (Eds.), *Neuropsychiatry of traumatic brain injury* (pp. 357–392). Washington DC: American Psychiatric Press.

Miller, L. (1992). Back to the future: Legal, vocational, and quality-of-life issues in the long-term adjustment of the brain-injured patient. *The Journal of Cognitive Rehabilitation,10*(5), 14–20.

Miller, L. (1996). Malingering in mild head injury and the post-concussion syndrome: Clinical, neuropsychological and forensic considerations. *The Journal of Cognitive Rehabilitation, 14*(4), 6–17.

Nies, K. J., & Sweet, J. J. (1994). Neuropsychological assessment and malingering: A critical review of past and present strategies. *Archives of Clinical Neuropsychology, 9*, 501–552.

Rimel, R. W. (1981). A prospective study of patients with central nervous system trauma. *Journal of Neurosurgical Nursing, 13*, 132–141.

Whitman, S., Coonley-Hoganson, R., & Desai, B. T. (1984). Comparative head trauma experiences in two socioeconomically different Chicago area communities—a population study. *American Journal of Epidemiology, 119*, 570–580.

Winograd, E. (1988). Some observations on prospective memory. In M. M. Gruneberg, P. E. Morris, & R. N. Sykes (Eds.), *Practical aspects of memory: Current research and issues* (Vol. 1, pp. 348–353). London: John Wiley and Sons.

Index

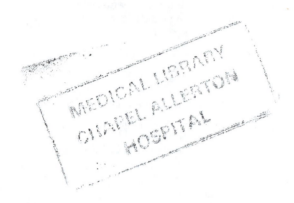